INSIDE THIS BOOK YOU WILL FIND :-

OVER 100 PLUS RECIPES, Grocery List for the Galveston DIET, Must-Have Kitchen TOOLS, Weekly Meal Plan TEMPLATE, Exercise and Movement for Sustainable Weight LOSS, Foods to AVOID And Many More, this are just the peak of it.

Galveston Diet

Cookbook

Transform Your Health: Recipes for Sustainable Weight Loss, Hormone Balance, and Vitality.

Author:- - SANDY P COLLETTE

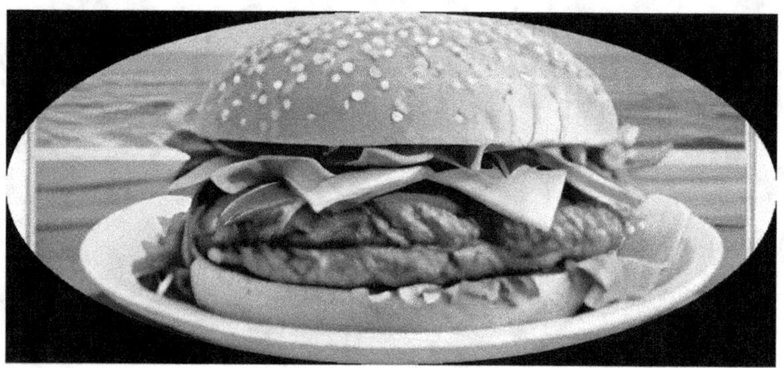

"Get your paperback copy today and receive a FREE
60-Day Meal Planner (exclusive bonus)! This
comprehensive planner is designed to help you
kickstart your weight loss journey and achieve your
goals. Don't miss out on this limited-time offer! Order
your paperback copy now and start planning your
path to a healthier, happier you!"

Gratitude Speech

"Dear amazing readers,
I am overwhelmed with gratitude and joy as I take a moment to express my heartfelt thanks to each and every one of you who has purchased my book. Your support means the world to me!

Your decision to invest in my work is a testament to the power of connection and community. It's a reminder that words have the ability to inspire, educate, and transform lives.

I am humbled by your trust in me and my writing. Your purchase is not just a transaction; it's a vote of confidence that fuels my passion to continue creating content that resonates with you.

Thank you for joining me on this journey. Thank you for being part of my story. I hope that my book has touched your heart, expanded your mind, or simply provided a moment of escape.

Your support is the wind in my sails, and I am forever grateful. Keep shining your light, and I will continue to do the same.

With deepest appreciation and love,
[SANDY P COLLETTE]"

Table of Contents

INTRODUCTION

<u>Welcome to the Galveston Diet Cookbook</u>

Dear Reader,
Welcome to the Galveston Diet Cookbook, a comprehensive guide to transforming your health through delicious recipes and science-backed nutritional principles.

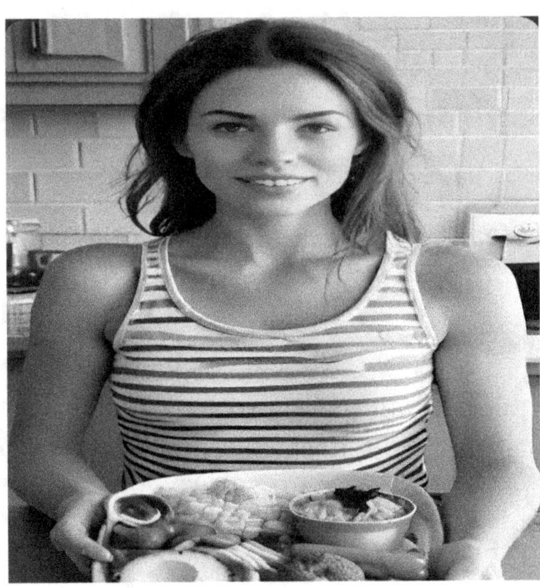

Whether you're looking to lose weight, achieve hormone balance, or simply enhance your vitality, this cookbook is designed to empower you on your journey to better health.

The Galveston Diet isn't just another fad; it's a well-researched approach developed by , to address the unique health needs of women's expertise in obstetrics and gynecology has led her to understand the profound impact that hormonal balance has on overall health, particularly in relation to weight management and energy levels.

The Science Behind the Galveston Diet: How It Works

At the heart of the Galveston Diet is a deep understanding of how hormones influence our bodies.

Hormonal imbalances, often exacerbated by stress, aging, and lifestyle factors, can lead to weight gain, fatigue, and a host of other health issues.

The Galveston Diet leverages specific dietary strategies to support hormonal equilibrium, promoting sustainable weight loss and increased vitality.

The Benefits of the Galveston Diet: Weight Loss, Hormone Balance, and Vitality

By following the Galveston Diet, many individuals have experienced not only significant weight loss but also improved mood, energy levels, and overall well-being.

The recipes in this cookbook are crafted with these benefits in mind, ensuring that each dish not only tastes great but also supports your body's natural processes.

How to Use This Cookbook

Navigating a new dietary approach can feel overwhelming, but this cookbook is designed to make it simple and enjoyable.

Here's how to get the most out of your Galveston Diet journey:

1. Understand the Principles: Take some time to familiarize yourself with the core principles of the Galveston Diet outlined in the following chapters. These principles will serve as the foundation for your meal planning and recipe selection.

2. Explore the Recipes: Dive into the diverse range of recipes carefully curated to align with the Galveston Diet principles. From hormone-balancing breakfasts to nourishing dinners and guilt-free desserts, each recipe is crafted to support your health goals without sacrificing flavor.

3. Prepare with Ease: Discover practical tips for meal preparation and efficient grocery shopping. Setting up your kitchen for success will streamline your cooking experience and make healthy eating a seamless part of your lifestyle.

4. Customize for Your Needs: While the Galveston Diet provides a structured framework, feel free to adapt recipes to suit your preferences and dietary requirements. Flexibility ensures that you can enjoy delicious meals while still achieving your health objectives.

Essential Tools and Ingredients for Success

Before you embark on your culinary journey, ensure you have the essential tools and ingredients recommended for preparing Galveston Diet recipes.

From basic kitchen utensils to key pantry staples, having these items on hand will facilitate smooth meal preparation and enhance your cooking experience.

In summary, the Galveston Diet Cookbook is more than just a collection of recipes—it's a guide to optimizing your health through mindful eating and balanced nutrition.

As you embark on this transformative journey, remember that every meal is an opportunity to nourish your body and embrace a healthier, happier lifestyle.

Here's to your health and wellness!

Warm regards,

Chapter 1: Understanding Hormones and Weight Loss

In this chapter, we delve into the intricate relationship between hormones and weight management.

Hormones play a crucial role in regulating metabolism, appetite, and fat storage.

Understanding how hormones influence these processes is key to achieving sustainable weight loss and overall well-being.

The Role of Hormones in Weight Management

Hormones act as chemical messengers that signal various bodily functions, including how our bodies store and utilize energy.

Key hormones involved in weight management include insulin, cortisol, leptin, and estrogen.

Each hormone plays a specific role in regulating appetite, metabolism, and fat distribution.

Common Hormonal Imbalances and Their Effects

Imbalances in hormones can disrupt these processes, leading to weight gain, fatigue, mood swings, and other health issues.

Common hormonal imbalances such as insulin resistance, thyroid dysfunction, and adrenal fatigue can significantly impact weight management efforts.

Recognizing the signs and symptoms of these imbalances is crucial for effective dietary and lifestyle interventions.

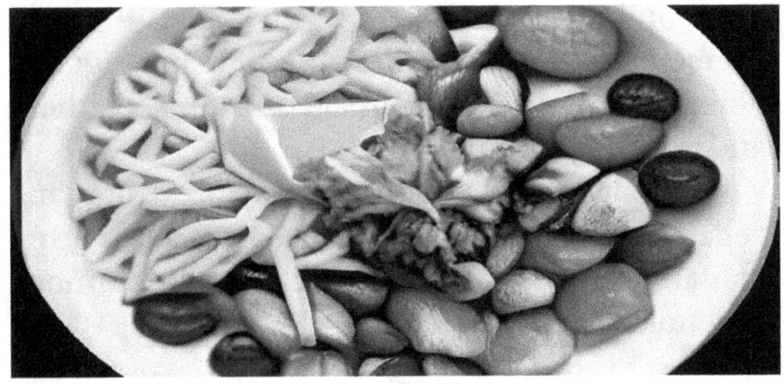

Chapter 2: The Role of Nutrition in Hormone Balance

Nutrition plays a pivotal role in supporting hormone balance and optimizing overall health. Certain nutrients and dietary patterns can help regulate hormone production and activity, promoting a balanced and efficient metabolism.

Key Nutrients for Hormone Health

- Omega-3 Fatty Acids: Found in fatty fish, flaxseeds, and walnuts, omega-3s help reduce inflammation and support hormone production.
- Vitamin D: Crucial for hormonal balance, vitamin D is synthesized in the skin through sunlight exposure and is also found in fortified foods and supplements.
- Fiber: Promotes gut health and helps regulate blood sugar levels, supporting insulin sensitivity and reducing cravings.
- Antioxidants: Found in colorful fruits and vegetables, antioxidants protect cells from oxidative stress and support overall hormone function.

- Protein: Essential for hormone production and muscle repair, lean protein sources include poultry, fish, tofu, and legumes.

Foods to Avoid

Certain foods can disrupt hormone balance and hinder weight loss efforts. These include:

- Refined Sugar: Causes spikes in blood sugar and insulin levels, contributing to insulin resistance.
- Processed Foods: Often high in unhealthy fats, sugars, and additives that can disrupt hormonal function.
- Trans Fats: Found in fried foods and packaged snacks, trans fats can increase inflammation and insulin resistance.
- Excessive Alcohol: Can interfere with hormone production and metabolism, leading to weight gain and hormonal imbalances.

Chapter 3: Setting Up Your Kitchen for Success

A well-equipped kitchen is essential for preparing nutritious meals that support the Galveston Diet principles. In this chapter, we explore the tools and organization strategies that will streamline your cooking experience and facilitate healthier eating habits.

Must-Have Kitchen Tools

Investing in quality kitchen tools can make meal preparation more efficient and enjoyable. Essential tools for your Galveston Diet kitchen include:

- Chef's Knife and Cutting Board: For chopping vegetables, fruits, and lean proteins.
- Non-Stick Cookware: Ensures minimal oil use and easy cleanup.
- Blender or Food Processor: Ideal for making smoothies, sauces, and soups.
- Measuring Cups and Spoons: Essential for portion control and accurate ingredient measurements.

- Steamer Basket: Preserves nutrients in vegetables during cooking.

Organizing Your Kitchen for Efficiency

Organizing your kitchen promotes healthier cooking habits and reduces meal preparation time. Tips for organizing your kitchen include:

- Clearing Clutter: Keep countertops clear of unnecessary items to create more workspace.
- Labeling Pantry Items: Use clear containers and labels to easily identify pantry staples like whole grains, nuts, and seeds.
- Meal Prep Stations: Designate areas for meal prep, such as a cutting board station or a smoothie-making corner.
- Refrigerator Organization: Store fresh produce at eye level for easy access and designate shelves for prepped meals and snacks.

Chapter 4: Essential Ingredients and Pantry Staples

Stocking your pantry with essential ingredients ensures you have everything you need to prepare nutritious Galveston Diet meals at home. These ingredients are not only versatile but also support hormone balance and overall health.

Key Ingredients for the Galveston Diet

- Lean Proteins: Chicken breast, turkey, lean cuts of beef, fish, tofu, and legumes.
- Whole Grains: Quinoa, brown rice, oats, and whole wheat pasta provide fiber and sustained energy.
- Healthy Fats: Avocado, nuts, seeds, olive oil, and fatty fish rich in omega-3s.
- Colorful Vegetables: Leafy greens, bell peppers, cruciferous vegetables (broccoli, cauliflower), and tomatoes are rich in antioxidants and fiber.

- Fresh Fruits: Berries, apples, citrus fruits, and bananas provide natural sweetness and essential vitamins.

Pantry Staples to Keep on Hand

Maintaining a well-stocked pantry ensures you can create nutritious meals without frequent trips to the grocery store. Essential pantry staples include:

- Canned Beans and Tomatoes: Versatile ingredients for soups, stews, and chili.
- Whole Grain Pasta and Rice: Quick-cooking options for hearty meals.
- Nuts and Seeds: Perfect for snacking and adding crunch to salads and oatmeal.
- Herbs and Spices: Enhance flavor without added salt or sugar.
- Broth and Stock: For adding depth to soups and sauces.

Chapter 5: Breakfast Recipes for Weight Loss and Hormone Balance

Start your day with nutritious and delicious breakfast options that support your weight loss goals and promote hormone balance.

These recipes are packed with essential nutrients, fiber, and healthy fats to keep you energized throughout the morning.

Recipe 1. Avocado and Egg Toast

Ingredients:
- 1 slice whole grain bread
- 1/2 avocado, mashed
- 1 egg, poached or fried
- Salt and pepper to taste
- Optional: sprinkle of red pepper flakes

Method:
1. Toast the whole grain bread until golden brown.
2. Spread mashed avocado evenly over the toast.
3. Top with a poached or fried egg.
4. Season with salt, pepper, and red pepper flakes if desired.

Cooking Time: 10 minutes
Nutritional Information:
- Calories: 300 kcal
- Protein: 15g
- Carbohydrates: 20g
- Fat: 18g
- Fiber: 7g

Recipe 2. Greek Yogurt Parfait

Ingredients:
- 1 cup plain Greek yogurt
- 1/2 cup mixed berries (such as strawberries, blueberries, raspberries)
- 1/4 cup granola
- Drizzle of honey or maple syrup (optional)

Method:
1. In a glass or bowl, layer Greek yogurt, mixed berries, and granola.
2. Repeat layers until ingredients are used up.
3. Drizzle with honey or maple syrup if desired.

Cooking Time: 5 minutes
Nutritional Information:
- Calories: 280 kcal
- Protein: 20g
- Carbohydrates: 35g
- Fat: 8g
- Fiber: 6g

Recipe 3. Chia Seed Pudding

Ingredients:
- 1/4 cup chia seeds
- 1 cup unsweetened almond milk (or any milk of choice)
- 1 tsp vanilla extract
- Fresh berries for topping

Method:
1. In a bowl, mix chia seeds, almond milk, and vanilla extract.
2. Stir well and let it sit for 10 minutes, then stir again to break up any clumps.
3. Cover and refrigerate overnight or for at least 2 hours until it thickens.
4. Serve chilled, topped with fresh berries.

Cooking Time: 10 minutes (plus chilling time)
Nutritional Information:
- Calories: 180 kcal
- Protein: 6g
- Carbohydrates: 20g
- Fat: 9g
- Fiber: 12g

Recipe 4. Spinach and Feta Omelet

Ingredients:
- 2 eggs
- Handful of fresh spinach leaves, chopped
- 2 tbsp crumbled feta cheese
- Salt and pepper to taste
- 1 tsp olive oil

Method:
1. In a bowl, whisk eggs until well combined.
2. Heat olive oil in a non-stick skillet over medium heat.
3. Add chopped spinach to the skillet and cook until wilted.
4. Pour beaten eggs over spinach, swirling to spread evenly.
5. Sprinkle feta cheese over the omelet.
6. Cook until eggs are set, then fold the omelet in half.
7. Season with salt and pepper, then serve hot.
Cooking Time: 15 minutes
Nutritional Information:
- Calories: 250 kcal
- Protein: 18g
- Carbohydrates: 3g
- Fat: 18g
- Fiber: 1g

Recipe 5. Mushroom and Tomato Scramble

Ingredients:
- 2 eggs
- 1/2 cup sliced mushrooms
- 1/2 cup cherry tomatoes, halved
- 1 tbsp chopped fresh parsley
- Salt and pepper to taste
- 1 tsp olive oil

Method:
1. Heat olive oil in a skillet over medium heat.
2. Add sliced mushrooms and cook until softened.
3. Add cherry tomatoes and cook for another 2-3 minutes until tomatoes are slightly softened.
4. In a bowl, whisk eggs with chopped parsley, salt, and pepper.
5. Pour eggs into the skillet with mushrooms and tomatoes.
6. Cook, stirring gently, until eggs are scrambled and fully cooked.
7. Serve hot, garnished with additional parsley if desired.

Cooking Time: 10 minutes
Nutritional Information:
- Calories: 200 kcal
- Protein: 14g

- Carbohydrates: 6g
- Fat: 12g
- Fiber: 2g

Recipe 6. Almond Butter Overnight Oats

Ingredients:
- 1/2 cup rolled oats
- 1 cup unsweetened almond milk (or any milk of choice)
- 1 tbsp almond butter
- 1 tbsp maple syrup or honey (optional)
- Sliced bananas for topping

Method:
1. In a jar or bowl, combine rolled oats, almond milk, almond butter, and maple syrup or honey.
2. Stir well until ingredients are fully mixed.
3. Cover and refrigerate overnight or for at least 4 hours.
4. Before serving, stir oats and add more almond milk if desired for desired consistency.
5. Top with sliced bananas before serving.

Cooking Time: 5 minutes (plus chilling time)
Nutritional Information:
- Calories: 320 kcal
- Protein: 9g
- Carbohydrates: 45g
- Fat: 12g
- Fiber: 7g

Recipe 7. Quinoa Breakfast Bowl

Ingredients:
- 1/2 cup cooked quinoa
- 1/2 cup plain Greek yogurt
- 1/4 cup mixed berries (such as strawberries, blueberries)
- 1 tbsp honey or maple syrup
- 1 tbsp chopped nuts (such as almonds or walnuts)

Method:
1. In a bowl, layer cooked quinoa and Greek yogurt.
2. Top with mixed berries, drizzle with honey or maple syrup, and sprinkle chopped nuts on top.
3. Serve immediately.

Cooking Time: 15 minutes (if quinoa needs to be cooked)
Nutritional Information:
- Calories: 300 kcal
- Protein: 15g
- Carbohydrates: 45g
- Fat: 8g
- Fiber: 5g

Recipe 8. Berry Antioxidant Smoothie

Ingredients:
- 1 cup mixed berries (strawberries, blueberries, raspberries)
- 1/2 cup plain Greek yogurt
- 1/2 cup unsweetened almond milk (or any milk of choice)
- 1 tbsp chia seeds
- Optional: honey or maple syrup for sweetness

Method:
1. Combine mixed berries, Greek yogurt, almond milk, and chia seeds in a blender.
2. Blend until smooth and creamy.
3. Add honey or maple syrup if additional sweetness is desired.
4. Pour into a glass and serve immediately.

Cooking Time: 5 minutes
Nutritional Information:
- Calories: 200 kcal
- Protein: 12g
- Carbohydrates: 30g
- Fat: 5g
- Fiber: 8g

Recipe 9. Almond Flour Pancakes

Ingredients:
- 1 cup almond flour
- 2 eggs
- 1/4 cup unsweetened almond milk (or any milk of choice)
- 1 tbsp maple syrup
- 1/2 tsp baking powder
- 1/2 tsp vanilla extract
- Pinch of salt

Method:
1. In a bowl, whisk together almond flour, eggs, almond milk, maple syrup, baking powder, vanilla extract, and salt until smooth.
2. Heat a non-stick skillet or griddle over medium heat.
3. Pour about 1/4 cup of batter onto the skillet for each pancake.
4. Cook until bubbles form on the surface, then flip and cook until golden brown on both sides.
5. Repeat with remaining batter.
6. Serve warm with fresh berries or a drizzle of honey.

Cooking Time: 15 minutes
Nutritional Information:

- Calories: 280 kcal
- Protein: 10g
- Carbohydrates: 15g
- Fat: 20g
- Fiber: 4g

Recipe 10. Sweet Potato Hash with Eggs

Ingredients:
- 1 medium sweet potato, peeled and diced
- 1/2 onion, diced
- 1 bell pepper, diced
- 2 eggs
- 1 tbsp olive oil
- Salt and pepper to taste
- Optional: sprinkle of paprika or cayenne pepper

Method:
1. Heat olive oil in a skillet over medium heat.
2. Add diced sweet potato and cook until slightly softened, about 5-7 minutes.
3. Add diced onion and bell pepper to the skillet and continue cooking until vegetables are tender.
4. Create two wells in the hash mixture and crack an egg into each well.
5. Cover the skillet and cook until eggs are cooked to your desired doneness.
6. Season with salt, pepper, and optional paprika or cayenne pepper.
7. Serve hot.

Cooking Time: 20 minutes
Nutritional Information:
- Calories: 320 kcal

- Protein: 14g
- Carbohydrates: 30g
- Fat: 16g
- Fiber: 6g

Recipe 11. Zucchini and Carrot Muffins

Ingredients:
- 1 cup grated zucchini
- 1/2 cup grated carrot
- 1 cup whole wheat flour (or almond flour for gluten-free option)
- 1/2 cup rolled oats
- 1/4 cup coconut sugar (or sweetener of choice)
- 1 tsp baking powder
- 1/2 tsp baking soda
- 1/2 tsp ground cinnamon
- 2 eggs
- 1/4 cup unsweetened applesauce
- 1/4 cup melted coconut oil
- 1 tsp vanilla extract
- Pinch of salt

Method:
1. Preheat the oven to 350°F (175°C). Line a muffin tin with paper liners or grease with coconut oil.
2. In a large bowl, combine grated zucchini and carrot.
3. In another bowl, whisk together flour, oats, coconut sugar, baking powder, baking soda, cinnamon, and salt.

4. In a separate bowl, beat eggs. Add applesauce, melted coconut oil, and vanilla extract, mixing well.

5. Pour wet ingredients into dry ingredients and stir until just combined.

6. Fold in grated zucchini and carrot until evenly distributed.

7. Spoon batter into muffin cups, filling each about 2/3 full.

8. Bake for 20-25 minutes, or until a toothpick inserted into the center comes out clean.

9. Allow muffins to cool in the tin for 5 minutes before transferring to a wire rack to cool completely.

Cooking Time: 30 minutes
Nutritional Information:
- Calories: 180 kcal
- Protein: 4g
- Carbohydrates: 22g
- Fat: 9g
- Fiber: 3g

Recipe 12. Cottage Cheese with Fresh Berries

Ingredients:
- 1/2 cup low-fat cottage cheese
- 1/2 cup mixed berries (such as strawberries, blueberries, raspberries)
- Drizzle of honey or maple syrup (optional)
- Fresh mint leaves for garnish

Method:
1. Spoon cottage cheese into a bowl or serving dish.
2. Top with mixed berries.
3. Drizzle with honey or maple syrup if desired.
4. Garnish with fresh mint leaves.

Preparation Time: 5 minutes
Nutritional Information:
- Calories: 120 kcal
- Protein: 12g
- Carbohydrates: 15g
- Fat: 2g
- Fiber: 3g

Recipe 13. Green Power Shake
Ingredients:
- 1 cup unsweetened almond milk (or any milk of choice)
- 1 cup fresh spinach leaves
- 1/2 avocado
- 1/2 banana
- 1 tbsp chia seeds
- Optional: honey or maple syrup for sweetness

Method:
1. In a blender, combine almond milk, spinach, avocado, banana, and chia seeds.
2. Blend until smooth and creamy.
3. Add honey or maple syrup if additional sweetness is desired.
4. Pour into a glass and serve immediately.

Preparation Time: 5 minutes
Nutritional Information:
- Calories: 250 kcal
- Protein: 8g
- Carbohydrates: 30g
- Fat: 14g
- Fiber: 10g

Recipe 14. Protein-Packed Omelet

Ingredients:
- 2 eggs
- 1/4 cup diced bell peppers (any color)
- 1/4 cup diced tomatoes
- 1/4 cup diced cooked chicken breast or tofu
- 1/4 cup shredded mozzarella cheese (or cheese of choice)
- Salt and pepper to taste
- 1 tsp olive oil

Method:
1. In a bowl, beat eggs until well combined.
2. Heat olive oil in a non-stick skillet over medium heat.
3. Add diced bell peppers and cook until slightly softened.
4. Add diced tomatoes and cooked chicken breast or tofu, cooking for another 2-3 minutes.
5. Pour beaten eggs into the skillet, swirling to spread evenly.
6. Cook until eggs are set around the edges.
7. Sprinkle shredded mozzarella cheese over one half of the omelet.
8. Fold the omelet in half over the cheese and cook for another minute until the cheese is melted.

9. Season with salt and pepper, then serve hot.

Cooking Time: 15 minutes
Nutritional Information:
- Calories: 300 kcal
- Protein: 25g
- Carbohydrates: 5g
- Fat: 20g
- Fiber: 2g

Recipe 15. Fresh Fruit and Nut Bowl

Ingredients:
- 1/2 cup mixed fresh fruits (such as berries, pineapple, mango)
- 1/4 cup plain Greek yogurt
- 2 tbsp mixed nuts (such as almonds, walnuts, pistachios)
- Drizzle of honey or maple syrup (optional)

Method:
1. Arrange mixed fresh fruits in a bowl.
2. Top with Greek yogurt and mixed nuts.
3. Drizzle with honey or maple syrup if desired.

Preparation Time: 5 minutes
Nutritional Information:
- Calories: 200 kcal
- Protein: 12g
- Carbohydrates: 25g
- Fat: 8g
- Fiber: 5g

Recipe 16. Flaxseed Banana Smoothie

Ingredients:
- 1 ripe banana
- 1 tbsp ground flaxseeds
- 1/2 cup plain Greek yogurt
- 1/2 cup unsweetened almond milk (or any milk of choice)
- 1 tsp honey or maple syrup (optional)
- Ice cubes (optional)

Method:
1. In a blender, combine ripe banana, ground flaxseeds, Greek yogurt, almond milk, and honey or maple syrup.
2. Add ice cubes if a colder smoothie is desired.
3. Blend until smooth and creamy.
4. Pour into a glass and serve immediately.

Preparation Time: 5 minutes
Nutritional Information:
- Calories: 220 kcal
- Protein: 10g
- Carbohydrates: 35g
- Fat: 5g
- Fiber: 6g

Recipe 17. Coconut Chia Pudding

Ingredients:
- 1/4 cup chia seeds
- 1 cup coconut milk (canned, full-fat)
- 1 tbsp maple syrup or honey
- 1/2 tsp vanilla extract
- Unsweetened shredded coconut for topping

Method:
1. In a bowl, mix chia seeds, coconut milk, maple syrup or honey, and vanilla extract.
2. Stir well and let it sit for 10 minutes, then stir again to break up any clumps.
3. Cover and refrigerate overnight or for at least 2 hours until it thickens.
4. Serve chilled, topped with unsweetened shredded coconut.

Preparation Time: 5 minutes (plus chilling time)
Nutritional Information:
- Calories: 280 kcal
- Protein: 6g
- Carbohydrates: 25g
- Fat: 18g
- Fiber: 10g

Recipe 18. Smoked Salmon and Avocado Plate

Ingredients:
- 2 oz smoked salmon
- 1/2 avocado, sliced
- 1 slice whole grain toast
- Fresh dill for garnish
- Lemon wedges (optional)

Method:
1. Toast the whole grain bread until golden brown.
2. Arrange smoked salmon and sliced avocado on the toast.
3. Garnish with fresh dill and serve with lemon wedges if desired.

Preparation Time: 5 minutes
Nutritional Information:
- Calories: 280 kcal
- Protein: 18g
- Carbohydrates: 20g
- Fat: 15g
- Fiber: 8g

Recipe 19. Mediterranean Quinoa Salad

Ingredients:
- 1 cup cooked quinoa
- 1 cup cherry tomatoes, halved
- 1/2 cucumber, diced
- 1/4 cup Kalamata olives, sliced
- 1/4 cup red onion, thinly sliced
- 1/4 cup crumbled feta cheese
- 2 tbsp fresh parsley, chopped
- Juice of 1 lemon
- 2 tbsp extra virgin olive oil
- Salt and pepper to taste

Method:
1. In a large bowl, combine cooked quinoa, cherry tomatoes, cucumber, Kalamata olives, red onion, feta cheese, and parsley.
2. Drizzle lemon juice and olive oil over the salad.
3. Season with salt and pepper, toss gently to combine.
4. Serve chilled.

Preparation Time: 15 minutes
Nutritional Information:
- Calories: 300 kcal
- Protein: 8g
- Carbohydrates: 30g
- Fat: 18g

- Fiber: 5g

Recipe 20. Grilled Chicken and Avocado Salad

Ingredients:
- 4 oz grilled chicken breast, sliced
- 1 avocado, sliced
- 2 cups mixed salad greens
- 1/2 cup cherry tomatoes, halved
- 1/4 cup cucumber, sliced
- 1/4 cup red bell pepper, sliced
- 2 tbsp balsamic vinaigrette dressing
- Salt and pepper to taste

Method:
1. Arrange mixed salad greens on a plate.
2. Top with grilled chicken breast, avocado slices, cherry tomatoes, cucumber, and red bell pepper.
3. Drizzle balsamic vinaigrette dressing over the salad.
4. Season with salt and pepper, toss gently to combine.

Preparation Time: 20 minutes
Nutritional Information:
- Calories: 350 kcal
- Protein: 30g
- Carbohydrates: 15g
- Fat: 20g
- Fiber: 8g

Recipe 21. Turkey and Hummus Wrap

Ingredients:
- 4 oz sliced turkey breast
- 2 tbsp hummus
- 1 whole wheat or gluten-free wrap
- 1/4 cup baby spinach leaves
- 1/4 cup shredded carrots
- 1/4 cup cucumber, thinly sliced
- Salt and pepper to taste

Method:
1. Spread hummus evenly over the wrap.
2. Layer sliced turkey breast, baby spinach leaves, shredded carrots, and cucumber slices on top.
3. Season with salt and pepper.
4. Roll up the wrap tightly, slice in half if desired, and serve.

Preparation Time: 10 minutes
Nutritional Information:
- Calories: 300 kcal
- Protein: 25g
- Carbohydrates: 25g
- Fat: 12g
- Fiber: 8g

Recipe 22. Roasted Beet and Goat Cheese Salad

Ingredients:
- 2 medium beets, roasted and sliced
- 2 cups mixed salad greens
- 1/4 cup crumbled goat cheese
- 1/4 cup walnuts, toasted
- 2 tbsp balsamic vinaigrette dressing
- Salt and pepper to taste

Method:
1. Preheat the oven to 400°F (200°C). Wrap beets in aluminum foil and roast for 45-60 minutes until tender. Let cool, then peel and slice.
2. Arrange mixed salad greens on a plate.
3. Top with roasted beet slices, crumbled goat cheese, and toasted walnuts.
4. Drizzle balsamic vinaigrette dressing over the salad.
5. Season with salt and pepper, toss gently to combine.

Preparation Time: 15 minutes (plus roasting time for beets)
Nutritional Information:
- Calories: 280 kcal
- Protein: 10g
- Carbohydrates: 20g

- Fat: 18g
- Fiber: 5g

Recipe 23. Lentil and Spinach Salad
Ingredients:
- 1 cup cooked lentils
- 2 cups fresh spinach leaves
- 1/4 cup cherry tomatoes, halved
- 1/4 cup cucumber, diced
- 1/4 cup red onion, thinly sliced
- 2 tbsp crumbled feta cheese
- 2 tbsp lemon juice
- 1 tbsp extra virgin olive oil
- Salt and pepper to taste

Method:
1. In a large bowl, combine cooked lentils, spinach leaves, cherry tomatoes, cucumber, red onion, and crumbled feta cheese.
2. Drizzle lemon juice and olive oil over the salad.
3. Season with salt and pepper, toss gently to combine.
4. Serve chilled or at room temperature.

Preparation Time: 15 minutes
Nutritional Information:
- Calories: 250 kcal
- Protein: 15g
- Carbohydrates: 30g
- Fat: 8g
- Fiber: 10g

Recipe 24. Salmon and Asparagus Salad
Ingredients:
- 4 oz grilled or baked salmon filet
- 1 cup asparagus spears, grilled or roasted
- 2 cups mixed salad greens
- 1/4 cup cherry tomatoes, halved
- 1/4 cup cucumber, sliced
- 2 tbsp lemon dill dressing
- Salt and pepper to taste

Method:
1. Grill or bake salmon filet until cooked through.
2. Grill or roast asparagus until tender-crisp.
3. Arrange mixed salad greens on a plate.
4. Top with grilled salmon, asparagus spears, cherry tomatoes, and cucumber slices.
5. Drizzle lemon dill dressing over the salad.
6. Season with salt and pepper, toss gently to combine.

Preparation Time: 20 minutes
Nutritional Information:
- Calories: 320 kcal
- Protein: 30g
- Carbohydrates: 15g
- Fat: 18g
- Fiber: 5g

Recipe 25. Stuffed Portobello Mushrooms

Ingredients:
- 4 large Portobello mushrooms
- 1 cup quinoa, cooked
- 1/2 cup cherry tomatoes, diced
- 1/2 cup baby spinach, chopped
- 1/4 cup crumbled feta cheese
- 2 tbsp balsamic glaze
- Salt and pepper to taste

Method:
1. Preheat the oven to 400°F (200°C). Remove stems from Portobello mushrooms and gently scrape out the gills.
2. In a bowl, combine cooked quinoa, cherry tomatoes, baby spinach, and crumbled feta cheese.
3. Season with salt and pepper.
4. Spoon quinoa mixture into Portobello mushroom caps, pressing gently to pack.
5. Place stuffed mushrooms on a baking sheet and bake for 20 minutes, or until mushrooms are tender.
6. Drizzle with balsamic glaze before serving.

Preparation Time: 30 minutes
Nutritional Information:

- Calories: 280 kcal
- Protein: 15g
- Carbohydrates: 35g
- Fat: 10g
- Fiber: 8g

Recipe 26. Tuna Salad Lettuce Wraps

Ingredients:
- 1 can (5 oz) tuna in water, drained
- 1/4 cup plain Greek yogurt
- 1 tbsp Dijon mustard
- 1/4 cup celery, diced
- 1/4 cup red onion, diced
- Salt and pepper to taste
- Butter lettuce leaves for wrapping

Method:
1. In a bowl, combine drained tuna, Greek yogurt, Dijon mustard, celery, and red onion.
2. Season with salt and pepper.
3. Spoon tuna salad into butter lettuce leaves.
4. Roll up lettuce leaves and secure with toothpicks if needed.
5. Serve immediately.

Preparation Time: 10 minutes
Nutritional Information:
- Calories: 200 kcal
- Protein: 25g
- Carbohydrates: 5g
- Fat: 8g
- Fiber: 2g

Recipe 27. Chicken and Veggie Stir-Fry

Ingredients:
- 4 oz chicken breast, sliced
- 1 cup broccoli florets
- 1/2 cup bell peppers, sliced
- 1/2 cup snap peas
- 1/4 cup carrots, sliced
- 2 tbsp soy sauce (low sodium)
- 1 tbsp hoisin sauce
- 1 clove garlic, minced
- 1 tsp ginger, minced
- 1 tbsp olive oil
- Sesame seeds for garnish (optional)
- Cooked brown rice or quinoa (optional)

Method:
1. Heat olive oil in a large skillet or wok over medium-high heat.
2. Add chicken breast slices and cook until browned and cooked through, about 5-7 minutes. Remove from the skillet and set aside.
3. In the same skillet, add broccoli florets, bell peppers, snap peas, and carrots. Stir-fry for 3-4 minutes until vegetables are tender-crisp.
4. Add minced garlic and ginger, stir-fry for another 30 seconds until fragrant.

5. Return cooked chicken breast slices to the skillet.

6. Add soy sauce and hoisin sauce, toss everything together until well combined and heated through.

7. Remove from heat and garnish with sesame seeds if desired.

8. Serve stir-fry alone or over cooked brown rice or quinoa.

Preparation Time: 25 minutes
Nutritional Information:
- Calories: 350 kcal
- Protein: 30g
- Carbohydrates: 25g
- Fat: 15g
- Fiber: 6g

Recipe 28. Quinoa and Black Bean Salad

Ingredients:
- 1 cup quinoa, cooked
- 1 can (15 oz) black beans, drained and rinsed
- 1 cup corn kernels (fresh or frozen, thawed)
- 1/2 cup cherry tomatoes, halved
- 1/4 cup red onion, finely chopped
- 1/4 cup fresh cilantro, chopped
- Juice of 1 lime
- 2 tbsp olive oil
- Salt and pepper to taste

Method:
1. In a large bowl, combine cooked quinoa, black beans, corn kernels, cherry tomatoes, red onion, and fresh cilantro.
2. In a small bowl, whisk together lime juice, olive oil, salt, and pepper.
3. Pour the dressing over the quinoa mixture and toss gently to combine.
4. Adjust seasoning if needed.
5. Serve chilled or at room temperature.

Preparation Time: 20 minutes
Nutritional Information:
- Calories: 320 kcal
- Protein: 12g

- Carbohydrates: 50g
- Fat: 8g
- Fiber: 10g

Recipe 29. Cauliflower Rice Bowl

Ingredients:
- 1 small head cauliflower, grated into rice-like texture
- 4 oz cooked chicken breast, diced
- 1/2 cup bell peppers, diced
- 1/2 cup cherry tomatoes, halved
- 1/4 cup black olives, sliced
- 2 tbsp pesto sauce
- Salt and pepper to taste

Method:
1. Heat a large skillet over medium heat.
2. Add grated cauliflower rice and cook for 5-7 minutes, stirring occasionally, until tender.
3. Add diced chicken breast, bell peppers, cherry tomatoes, and black olives to the skillet.
4. Cook for another 3-4 minutes until vegetables are heated through and chicken is warmed.
5. Stir in pesto sauce and toss everything together until well combined.
6. Season with salt and pepper.
7. Serve the cauliflower rice bowl warm.

Preparation Time: 20 minutes
Nutritional Information:
- Calories: 280 kcal

- Protein: 25g
- Carbohydrates: 15g
- Fat: 12g
- Fiber: 8g

Recipe 30. Zoodle (Zucchini Noodle) Salad

Ingredients:
- 2 large zucchinis, spiralized into noodles
- 1/2 cup cherry tomatoes, halved
- 1/4 cup red onion, thinly sliced
- 1/4 cup crumbled feta cheese
- 2 tbsp fresh basil leaves, chopped
- 2 tbsp balsamic vinaigrette dressing
- Salt and pepper to taste

Method:
1. In a large bowl, combine zucchini noodles, cherry tomatoes, red onion, crumbled feta cheese, and fresh basil leaves.
2. Drizzle balsamic vinaigrette dressing over the salad.
3. Season with salt and pepper, toss gently to combine.
4. Serve zoodle salad chilled.

Preparation Time: 15 minutes
Nutritional Information:
- Calories: 180 kcal
- Protein: 8g
- Carbohydrates: 15g
- Fat: 10g
- Fiber: 5g

Recipe 31. Greek Chickpea Salad

Ingredients:
- 1 can (15 oz) chickpeas, drained and rinsed
- 1/2 cucumber, diced
- 1/2 cup cherry tomatoes, halved
- 1/4 cup red onion, finely chopped
- 1/4 cup Kalamata olives, sliced
- 1/4 cup crumbled feta cheese
- 2 tbsp fresh parsley, chopped
- Juice of 1 lemon
- 2 tbsp extra virgin olive oil
- Salt and pepper to taste

Method:
1. In a large bowl, combine chickpeas, cucumber, cherry tomatoes, red onion, Kalamata olives, crumbled feta cheese, and fresh parsley.
2. Drizzle lemon juice and olive oil over the salad.
3. Season with salt and pepper, toss gently to combine.
4. Serve Greek chickpea salad chilled.

Preparation Time: 15 minutes
Nutritional Information:
- Calories: 280 kcal
- Protein: 12g
- Carbohydrates: 30g

- Fat: 12g
- Fiber: 8g

Recipe 32. Shrimp and Avocado Salad
Ingredients:
- 4 oz cooked shrimp, peeled and deveined
- 1 avocado, diced
- 2 cups mixed salad greens
- 1/2 cup cherry tomatoes, halved
- 1/4 cup cucumber, sliced
- 2 tbsp cilantro leaves, chopped
- 2 tbsp lime juice
- 1 tbsp olive oil
- Salt and pepper to taste

Method:
1. In a large bowl, combine mixed salad greens, cooked shrimp, avocado, cherry tomatoes, cucumber, and cilantro leaves.
2. Drizzle lime juice and olive oil over the salad.
3. Season with salt and pepper, toss gently to combine.
4. Serve shrimp and avocado salad chilled.

Preparation Time: 15 minutes
Nutritional Information:
- Calories: 320 kcal
- Protein: 25g
- Carbohydrates: 15g
- Fat: 18g
- Fiber: 8g

Recipe 33. Vegan Buddha Bowl

Ingredients:
- 1 cup cooked quinoa
- 1/2 cup cooked chickpeas
- 1/2 cup roasted sweet potatoes, cubed
- 1/2 cup steamed broccoli florets
- 1/4 cup shredded purple cabbage
- 1/4 cup shredded carrots
- 2 tbsp tahini dressing (tahini, lemon juice, garlic, water)
- Salt and pepper to taste

Method:
1. Arrange cooked quinoa, chickpeas, roasted sweet potatoes, steamed broccoli florets, shredded purple cabbage, and shredded carrots in a bowl.
2. Drizzle tahini dressing over the bowl.
3. Season with salt and pepper, toss gently to combine.
4. Serve a vegan Buddha bowl warm or at room temperature.

Preparation Time: 30 minutes
Nutritional Information:
- Calories: 380 kcal
- Protein: 15g

- Carbohydrates: 50g
- Fat: 15g
- Fiber: 12g

Recipe 34. Spinach and Quinoa Stuffed Peppers

Ingredients:
- 4 bell peppers, halved and seeds removed
- 1 cup quinoa, cooked
- 1 cup baby spinach leaves, chopped
- 1/2 cup cherry tomatoes, diced
- 1/4 cup red onion, finely chopped
- 1/4 cup crumbled feta cheese
- 2 tbsp fresh basil leaves, chopped
- Salt and pepper to taste

Method:
1. Preheat the oven to 375°F (190°C).
2. In a large bowl, combine cooked quinoa, chopped baby spinach, cherry tomatoes, red onion, crumbled feta cheese, and fresh basil leaves.
3. Season with salt and pepper.
4. Stuffed bell pepper halves with quinoa mixture.
5. Place stuffed peppers in a baking dish and cover with foil.
6. Bake for 25-30 minutes until peppers are tender and filling is heated through.
7. Serve spinach and quinoa stuffed peppers warm.

Preparation Time: 40 minutes

Nutritional Information:
- Calories: 250 kcal
- Protein: 10g
- Carbohydrates: 35g
- Fat: 8g
- Fiber: 8g

Recipe 35. Sweet Potato and Black Bean Tacos

Ingredients:
- 4 small corn or flour tortillas
- 1 cup sweet potatoes, diced and roasted
- 1 can (15 oz) black beans, drained and rinsed
- 1/2 cup red cabbage, shredded
- 1/4 cup fresh cilantro leaves
- 1/4 cup salsa (mild, medium, or hot as per preference)
- Lime wedges for serving
- Salt and pepper to taste

Method:
1. Warm tortillas according to package instructions.
2. Fill each tortilla with roasted sweet potatoes, black beans, shredded red cabbage, and fresh cilantro leaves.
3. Drizzle salsa over the tacos.
4. Season with salt and pepper.
5. Serve sweet potato and black bean tacos with lime wedges on the side.

Preparation Time: 30 minutes
Nutritional Information:
- Calories: 280 kcal
- Protein: 10g

- Carbohydrates: 50g
- Fat: 5g
- Fiber: 10g

Recipe 36. Thai Chicken Salad

Ingredients:
- 4 oz grilled chicken breast, sliced
- 2 cups mixed salad greens
- 1/2 cup mango, diced
- 1/4 cup red bell pepper, sliced
- 1/4 cup cucumber, sliced
- 1/4 cup red onion, thinly sliced
- 2 tbsp fresh cilantro leaves, chopped
- 2 tbsp Thai peanut dressing
- Salt and pepper to taste

Method:
1. Arrange mixed salad greens on a plate.
2.Top with grilled chicken breast slices, diced mango, red bell pepper, cucumber slices, red onion, and fresh cilantro leaves.

3. Drizzle Thai peanut dressing over the salad.
4. Season with salt and pepper, toss gently to combine.
5. Serve Thai chicken salad chilled.

Preparation Time: 20 minutes
Nutritional Information:
- Calories: 320 kcal
- Protein: 30g

- Carbohydrates: 20g
- Fat: 15g
- Fiber: 5g

Recipe 37. Roasted Vegetable and Hummus Wrap

Ingredients:
- 1 whole wheat or gluten-free wrap
- 1/4 cup hummus
- 1/2 cup mixed roasted vegetables (zucchini, bell peppers, eggplant, etc.)
- Handful of mixed salad greens
- Salt and pepper to taste

Method:
1. Spread hummus evenly over the wrap.
2. Layer mixed roasted vegetables and mixed salad greens on top.
3. Season with salt and pepper.
4. Roll up the wrap tightly, slice in half if desired, and serve.

Preparation Time: 15 minutes
Nutritional Information:
- Calories: 250 kcal
- Protein: 8g
- Carbohydrates: 35g
- Fat: 10g
- Fiber: 8g

Recipe 38. Baked Salmon with Lemon and Herbs

Ingredients:
- 4 oz salmon filet
- 1 tbsp olive oil
- 1 tbsp fresh lemon juice
- 1 tsp lemon zest
- 1 clove garlic, minced
- 1 tsp fresh dill, chopped
- Salt and pepper to taste

Method:
1. Preheat the oven to 400°F (200°C).
2. Place salmon filet on a baking sheet lined with parchment paper.
3. In a small bowl, whisk together olive oil, lemon juice, lemon zest, minced garlic, chopped dill, salt, and pepper.
4. Pour the mixture over the salmon filet, spreading it evenly.
5. Bake for 12-15 minutes until salmon is cooked through and flakes easily with a fork.
6. Remove from the oven and let rest for a few minutes before serving.

Preparation Time: 20 minutes
Nutritional Information:
- Calories: 300 kcal

- Protein: 30g
- Carbohydrates: 2g
- Fat: 20g
- Fiber: 0g

Recipe 39. Garlic Herb Roasted Chicken

Ingredients:
- 4 oz chicken breast
- 1 tbsp olive oil
- 1 clove garlic, minced
- 1 tsp fresh thyme, chopped
- 1 tsp fresh rosemary, chopped
- Salt and pepper to taste

Method:
1. Preheat the oven to 400°F (200°C).
2. In a small bowl, combine olive oil, minced garlic, chopped thyme, chopped rosemary, salt, and pepper.
3. Place chicken breast in a baking dish or on a baking sheet lined with parchment paper.
4. Brush the garlic herb mixture over the chicken breast, coating it evenly.
5. Bake for 20-25 minutes until chicken is cooked through and juices run clear.
6. Remove from the oven and let rest for a few minutes before serving.

Preparation Time: 30 minutes
Nutritional Information:
- Calories: 280 kcal
- Protein: 30g

- Carbohydrates: 1g
- Fat: 16g
- Fiber: 0g

Recipe 40. Stuffed Bell Peppers

Ingredients:
- 4 bell peppers, tops removed and seeds removed
- 1 cup quinoa, cooked
- 1 can (15 oz) black beans, drained and rinsed
- 1 cup corn kernels (fresh or frozen, thawed)
- 1/2 cup cherry tomatoes, diced
- 1/4 cup red onion, finely chopped
- 1/4 cup shredded cheddar cheese (optional)
- 2 tbsp fresh cilantro leaves, chopped
- 1 tsp ground cumin
- 1 tsp chili powder
- Salt and pepper to taste

Method:
1. Preheat the oven to 375°F (190°C).
2. In a large bowl, combine cooked quinoa, black beans, corn kernels, cherry tomatoes, red onion, shredded cheddar cheese (if using), fresh cilantro leaves, ground cumin, chili powder, salt, and pepper.
3. Stuff bell peppers with quinoa mixture, pressing gently to pack.
4. Place stuffed peppers upright in a baking dish.
5. Cover with foil and bake for 25-30 minutes until peppers are tender.

6. Remove foil and bake for an additional 5 minutes to melt cheese if using.
7. Serve stuffed bell peppers warm.

Preparation Time: 45 minutes
Nutritional Information:
- Calories: 320 kcal
- Protein: 15g
- Carbohydrates: 55g
- Fat: 5g
- Fiber: 12g

Recipe 41. Zucchini Noodles with Pesto
Ingredients:
- 2 large zucchinis, spiralized into noodles
- 1/4 cup homemade or store-bought pesto sauce
- 1/4 cup cherry tomatoes, halved
- 1/4 cup toasted pine nuts
- Fresh basil leaves for garnish
- Salt and pepper to taste

Method:
1. Heat a large skillet over medium heat.
2. Add spiralized zucchini noodles and cook for 3-4 minutes until tender-crisp.
3. Add pesto sauce to the skillet and toss with zucchini noodles until well combined.
4. Stir in cherry tomatoes and toasted pine nuts.
5. Season with salt and pepper.
6. Remove from heat and garnish with fresh basil leaves.
7. Serve zucchini noodles with pesto warm.

Preparation Time: 15 minutes
Nutritional Information:
- Calories: 250 kcal
- Protein: 8g
- Carbohydrates: 12g
- Fat: 20g
- Fiber: 4g

Recipe 42. Grilled Shrimp Skewers

Ingredients:
- 8 oz large shrimp, peeled and deveined
- 1 tbsp olive oil
- 1 clove garlic, minced
- 1 tsp smoked paprika
- 1/2 tsp ground cumin
- Salt and pepper to taste
- Lemon wedges for serving

Method:
1. Preheat the grill or grill pan over medium-high heat.
2. In a bowl, combine olive oil, minced garlic, smoked paprika, ground cumin, salt, and pepper.
3. Add shrimp to the bowl and toss to coat evenly.
4. Thread shrimp on skewers.
5. Grill shrimp skewers for 2-3 minutes per side until shrimp are pink and opaque.
6. Remove from the grill and serve with lemon wedges.

Preparation Time: 15 minutes
Nutritional Information:
- Calories: 180 kcal
- Protein: 25g
- Carbohydrates: 2g

- Fat: 8g
- Fiber: 0g

Recipe 43. Beef and Broccoli Stir-Fry

Ingredients:
- 4 oz beef sirloin, thinly sliced
- 2 cups broccoli florets
- 1/2 cup bell peppers, sliced
- 1/4 cup sliced carrots
- 1/4 cup soy sauce (low sodium)
- 1 tbsp oyster sauce
- 1 tbsp hoisin sauce
- 1 clove garlic, minced
- 1 tsp ginger, minced
- 1 tbsp olive oil
- Cooked brown rice for serving

Method:
1. Heat olive oil in a large skillet or wok over medium-high heat.
2. Add thinly sliced beef sirloin and cook until browned, about 3-4 minutes. Remove from the skillet and set aside.
3. In the same skillet, add broccoli florets, bell peppers, sliced carrots, minced garlic, and minced ginger.
4. Stir-fry for 4-5 minutes until vegetables are tender-crisp.
5. Return cooked beef sirloin to the skillet.

6. Add soy sauce, oyster sauce, and hoisin sauce, tossing everything together until well combined and heated through.
7. Serve beef and broccoli stir-fry over cooked brown rice.

Preparation Time: 25 minutes
Nutritional Information:
- Calories: 380 kcal
- Protein: 30g
- Carbohydrates: 30g
- Fat: 15g
- Fiber: 6g

Recipe 44. Turkey Meatballs in Tomato Sauce

Ingredients:
- 8 oz ground turkey
- 1/4 cup breadcrumbs (whole wheat or gluten-free)
- 1/4 cup grated Parmesan cheese
- 1 egg
- 1 clove garlic, minced
- 1 tsp Italian seasoning
- Salt and pepper to taste
- 1 tbsp olive oil
- 1 can (15 oz) tomato sauce
- Fresh basil leaves for garnish

Method:
1. Preheat the oven to 400°F (200°C).
2. In a bowl, combine ground turkey, breadcrumbs, grated Parmesan cheese, egg, minced garlic, Italian seasoning, salt, and pepper. Mix until well combined.
3. Shape mixture into meatballs (about 1 inch in diameter).
4. Heat olive oil in a large skillet over medium-high heat.
5. Add meatballs to the skillet and cook until browned on all sides, about 5 minutes.

6. Transfer meatballs to a baking dish and pour tomato sauce over them.
7. Bake meatballs in the
oven for 15-20 minutes until fully cooked.

8. Garnish with fresh basil leaves before serving.

Preparation Time: 35 minutes
Nutritional Information:
- Calories: 280 kcal
- Protein: 25g
- Carbohydrates: 15g
- Fat: 12g
- Fiber: 3g

Recipe 45. Cod with Tomato Basil Sauce

Ingredients:
- 4 oz cod filet
- 1 tbsp olive oil
- 1 clove garlic, minced
- 1 cup cherry tomatoes, halved
- 1/4 cup fresh basil leaves, chopped
- 1 tbsp balsamic vinegar
- Salt and pepper to taste

Method:
1. Preheat the oven to 375°F (190°C).
2. Heat olive oil in a skillet over medium heat.
3. Add minced garlic and cook until fragrant, about 1 minute.
4. Add cherry tomatoes and cook until they begin to soften, about 3-4 minutes.
5. Stir in fresh basil leaves and balsamic vinegar, cook for an additional 2 minutes.
6. Place cod filet in a baking dish and pour tomato basil sauce over it.
7. Season with salt and pepper.
8. Bake for 15-20 minutes until cod is cooked through and flakes easily with a fork.
9. Serve cod with tomato basil sauce warm.

Preparation Time: 25 minutes

Nutritional Information:
- Calories: 220 kcal
- Protein: 25g
- Carbohydrates: 10g
- Fat: 10g
- Fiber: 3g

Recipe 46. Lemon Garlic Shrimp Pasta (Zoodles)

Ingredients:
- 2 large zucchinis, spiralized into noodles
- 8 oz shrimp, peeled and deveined
- 1 tbsp olive oil
- 2 cloves garlic, minced
- Juice of 1 lemon
- Zest of 1 lemon
- 1/4 cup grated Parmesan cheese
- Salt and pepper to taste
- Fresh parsley for garnish

Method:
1. Heat olive oil in a large skillet over medium heat.
2. Add minced garlic and cook until fragrant, about 1 minute.
3. Add shrimp and cook until pink and opaque, about 2-3 minutes per side.
4. Stir in lemon juice and lemon zest.
5. Add spiralized zucchini noodles to the skillet and cook for 2-3 minutes until tender-crisp.
6. Sprinkle grated Parmesan cheese, salt, and pepper.
7. Toss everything together until well combined.
8. Garnish with fresh parsley and serve lemon garlic shrimp pasta warm.

Preparation Time: 20 minutes
Nutritional Information:
- **Calories:** 280 kcal
- **Protein:** 25g
- **Carbohydrates:** 10g
- **Fat:** 15g
- **Fiber:** 4g

Recipe 47. Cauliflower Crust Pizza

Ingredients:
- 1 small head cauliflower, grated into rice-like texture
- 1/4 cup grated Parmesan cheese
- 1/4 cup shredded mozzarella cheese
- 1 egg, beaten
- 1 tsp Italian seasoning
- 1/2 cup tomato sauce
- 1/2 cup shredded mozzarella cheese (for topping)
- Various toppings (e.g., bell peppers, onions, mushrooms, olives, etc.)
- Salt and pepper to taste

Method:
1. Preheat the oven to 425°F (220°C).
2. Steam grated cauliflower until tender, about 5-7 minutes. Let cool and squeeze out excess moisture using a clean kitchen towel.
3. In a bowl, combine steamed cauliflower, grated Parmesan cheese, shredded mozzarella cheese, beaten egg, Italian seasoning, salt, and pepper.
4. Line a baking sheet with parchment paper and spread cauliflower mixture into a thin, even layer.
5. Bake for 15-20 minutes until golden brown and crispy.

6. Remove from the oven and spread tomato sauce over the crust.

7. Top with shredded mozzarella cheese and desired toppings.

8. Return to the oven and bake for an additional 10-12 minutes until the cheese is melted and bubbly.

9. Serve cauliflower crust pizza warm.

Preparation Time: 35 minutes
Nutritional Information:
- Calories: 250 kcal
- Protein: 15g
- Carbohydrates: 12g
- Fat: 15g
- Fiber: 5g

Recipe 48. Moroccan Chicken with Quinoa

Ingredients:
- 4 oz chicken breast, diced
- 1 tbsp olive oil
- 1 clove garlic, minced
- 1 tsp ground cumin
- 1/2 tsp ground cinnamon
- 1/2 tsp ground turmeric
- 1/2 tsp ground coriander
- 1/2 cup diced tomatoes
- 1/4 cup chicken broth
- 1/4 cup raisins
- 1 cup cooked quinoa
- Fresh cilantro for garnish
- Salt and pepper to taste

Method:
1. Heat olive oil in a skillet over medium heat.
2. Add diced chicken breast and cook until browned, about 5-7 minutes.
3. Stir in minced garlic, ground cumin, ground cinnamon, ground turmeric, and ground coriander.
4. Add diced tomatoes, chicken broth, and raisins. Cook for an additional 5 minutes until chicken is cooked through and sauce is thickened.
5. Serve Moroccan chicken over cooked quinoa.

6. Garnish with fresh cilantro and serve warm.

Preparation Time: 30 minutes
Nutritional Information:
- Calories: 350 kcal
- Protein: 30g
- Carbohydrates: 45g
- Fat: 8g
- Fiber: 6g

Recipe 49. Eggplant Parmesan (Baked)

Ingredients:
- 1 large eggplant, sliced into rounds
- 1/2 cup breadcrumbs (whole wheat or gluten-free)
- 1/4 cup grated Parmesan cheese
- 1 egg, beaten
- 1 cup tomato sauce
- 1/2 cup shredded mozzarella cheese
- Fresh basil leaves for garnish
- Salt and pepper to taste

Method:
1. Preheat the oven to 375°F (190°C).
2. In a shallow bowl, combine breadcrumbs and grated Parmesan cheese.
3. Dip eggplant slices in beaten egg, then coat with breadcrumb mixture.
4. Place breaded eggplant slices on a baking sheet lined with parchment paper.
5. Bake for 20-25 minutes until golden brown and crispy.
6. Remove from the oven and spread a thin layer of tomato sauce over each eggplant slice.
7. Top with shredded mozzarella cheese.

8. Return to the oven and bake for an additional 10-12 minutes until the cheese is melted and bubbly.

9. Garnish with fresh basil leaves and serve eggplant Parmesan warm.

Preparation Time: 40 minutes
Nutritional Information:
- Calories: 280 kcal
- Protein: 12g
- Carbohydrates: 30g
- Fat: 12g
- Fiber: 8g

Recipe 50. Pork Tenderloin with Roasted Vegetables

Ingredients:
- 4 oz pork tenderloin
- 1 tbsp olive oil
- 1 clove garlic, minced
- 1 tsp fresh rosemary, chopped
- 1 tsp fresh thyme, chopped
- 1 cup mixed vegetables (carrots, Brussels sprouts, bell peppers, etc.), diced
- Salt and pepper to taste

Method:
1. Preheat the oven to 400°F (200°C).
2. In a bowl, combine olive oil, minced garlic, chopped rosemary, chopped thyme, salt, and pepper.
3. Rub the mixture over the pork tenderloin.
4. Place pork tenderloin on a baking sheet lined with parchment paper.
5. Arrange mixed vegetables around the pork tenderloin.
6. Roast for 25-30 minutes until pork is cooked through and vegetables are tender.
7. Let pork rest for a few minutes before slicing.
8. Serve pork tenderloin with roasted vegetables warm.

Preparation Time: 35 minutes
Nutritional Information:
- Calories: 320 kcal
- Protein: 30g
- Carbohydrates: 20g
- Fat: 12g
- Fiber: 6g

Recipe 51. Chickpea and Spinach Curry

Ingredients:
- 1 can (15 oz) chickpeas, drained and rinsed
- 1 tbsp olive oil
- 1 onion, finely chopped
- 2 cloves garlic, minced
- 1 tsp ground cumin
- 1 tsp ground coriander
- 1 tsp ground turmeric
- 1/2 tsp ground cinnamon
- 1 can (14 oz) diced tomatoes
- 1/2 cup coconut milk
- 2 cups fresh spinach leaves
- Salt and pepper to taste
- Fresh cilantro for garnish

Method:
1. Heat olive oil in a large skillet over medium heat.
2. Add finely chopped onion and cook until softened, about 5 minutes.
3. Stir in minced garlic, ground cumin, ground coriander, ground turmeric, and ground cinnamon. Cook for an additional 1-2 minutes until fragrant.
4. Add diced tomatoes and coconut milk, stirring to combine.

5. Stir in chickpeas and bring to a simmer.
6. Add fresh spinach leaves and cook until wilted, about 2-3 minutes.
7. Season with salt and pepper.
8. Serve chickpea and spinach curry garnished with fresh cilantro.

Preparation Time: 30 minutes
Nutritional Information:
- Calories: 320 kcal
- Protein: 10g
- Carbohydrates: 40g
- Fat: 15g
- Fiber: 10g

Recipe 52. Lentil and Vegetable Soup

Ingredients:

- 1 cup lentils, rinsed and drained
- 1 tbsp olive oil
- 1 onion, finely chopped
- 2 cloves garlic, minced
- 2 carrots, diced
- 2 celery stalks, diced
- 1 can (14 oz) diced tomatoes
- 4 cups vegetable broth
- 1 tsp dried thyme
- 1 bay leaf
- 2 cups fresh spinach leaves
- Salt and pepper to taste

Method:
1. Heat olive oil in a large pot over medium heat.
2. Add finely chopped onion, minced garlic, diced carrots, and diced celery. Cook until vegetables are softened, about 5-7 minutes.
3. Stir in lentils, diced tomatoes, vegetable broth, dried thyme, and bay leaf.
4. Bring to a boil, then reduce heat and simmer for 25-30 minutes until lentils are tender.

5. Remove bay leaf and stir in fresh spinach leaves until wilted.
6. Season with salt and pepper.
7. Serve lentil and vegetable soup warm.

Preparation Time: 40 minutes
Nutritional Information:
- Calories: 280 kcal
- Protein: 15g
- Carbohydrates: 45g
- Fat: 6g
- Fiber: 15g

Recipe 53. Quinoa and Black Bean Stuffed Peppers

Ingredients:
- 4 bell peppers, tops removed and seeds removed
- 1 cup quinoa, cooked
- 1 can (15 oz) black beans, drained and rinsed
- 1/2 cup corn kernels (fresh or frozen, thawed)
- 1/2 cup diced tomatoes
- 1/4 cup red onion, finely chopped
- 1/4 cup shredded cheddar cheese (optional)
- 2 tbsp fresh cilantro leaves, chopped
- 1 tsp ground cumin
- 1 tsp chili powder
- Salt and pepper to taste

Method:
1. Preheat the oven to 375°F (190°C).
2. In a large bowl, combine cooked quinoa, black beans, corn kernels, diced tomatoes, red onion, shredded cheddar cheese (if using), fresh cilantro leaves, ground cumin, chili powder, salt, and pepper.
3. Stuff bell peppers with quinoa mixture, pressing gently to pack.
4. Place stuffed peppers upright in a baking dish.
5. Cover with foil and bake for 25-30 minutes until peppers are tender.

6. Remove foil and bake for an additional 5 minutes to melt cheese if using.
7. Serve stuffed bell peppers warm.

Preparation Time: 45 minutes
Nutritional Information:
- Calories: 320 kcal
- Protein: 15g
- Carbohydrates: 55g
- Fat: 5g
- Fiber: 12g

Recipe 54. Seared Tuna with Mango Salsa

Ingredients:
- 4 oz tuna steak
- 1 tbsp olive oil
- Salt and pepper to taste
- 1 ripe mango, diced
- 1/4 cup red onion, finely chopped
- 1/4 cup red bell pepper, diced
- 1/4 cup fresh cilantro, chopped
- Juice of 1 lime

Method:
1. Season tuna steak with salt and pepper.
2. Heat olive oil in a skillet over medium-high heat.
3. Sear tuna steak for 2-3 minutes per side, until desired doneness is reached.
4. In a bowl, combine diced mango, red onion, red bell pepper, fresh cilantro, and lime juice to make the mango salsa.
5. Serve seared tuna topped with mango salsa.

Preparation Time: 20 minutes
Nutritional Information:
- Calories: 350 kcal
- Protein: 30g
- Carbohydrates: 25g

- Fat: 12g
- Fiber: 3g

Recipe 55. Sweet Potato and Kale Hash

Ingredients:
- 1 large sweet potato, peeled and diced
- 1 tbsp olive oil
- 1 onion, finely chopped
- 2 cloves garlic, minced
- 2 cups fresh kale, chopped
- Salt and pepper to taste

Method:
1. Heat olive oil in a large skillet over medium heat.
2. Add diced sweet potato and cook for 10-12 minutes until tender.
3. Add finely chopped onion and minced garlic, cooking until onion is translucent, about 5 minutes.
4. Stir in fresh kale and cook until wilted, about 3-4 minutes.
5. Season with salt and pepper.
6. Serve sweet potato and kale hash warm.

Preparation Time: 25 minutes
Nutritional Information:
- Calories: 250 kcal
- Protein: 5g
- Carbohydrates: 45g

- Fat: 8g
- Fiber: 8g

Recipe 56. Tofu and Vegetable Stir-Fry

Ingredients:
- 8 oz firm tofu, cubed
- 1 tbsp sesame oil
- 1 clove garlic, minced
- 1 tsp fresh ginger, grated
- 1 cup broccoli florets
- 1 bell pepper, sliced
- 1 carrot, julienned
- 1/4 cup soy sauce or tamari
- 2 tbsp rice vinegar
- 1 tbsp honey or maple syrup
- 1 tbsp cornstarch mixed with 2 tbsp water (optional, for thickening)
- 2 green onions, sliced

Method:
1. Heat sesame oil in a large skillet or wok over medium-high heat.
2. Add cubed tofu and cook until golden brown on all sides, about 5-7 minutes. Remove tofu from the skillet and set aside.
3. In the same skillet, add minced garlic and grated ginger, cooking for 1 minute until fragrant.

4. Add broccoli florets, bell pepper slices, and julienned carrot, stir-frying for 5-7 minutes until vegetables are tender-crisp.
5. In a small bowl, mix soy sauce or tamari, rice vinegar, and honey or maple syrup.
6. Return tofu to the skillet and pour sauce over the stir-fry. If a thicker sauce is desired, add cornstarch mixture.
7. Stir everything together until well coated and heated through, about 2-3 minutes.
8. Garnish with sliced green onions and serve tofu and vegetable stir-fry warm.

Preparation Time: 30 minutes
Nutritional Information:
- Calories: 320 kcal
- Protein: 15g
- Carbohydrates: 30g
- Fat: 15g
- Fiber: 6g

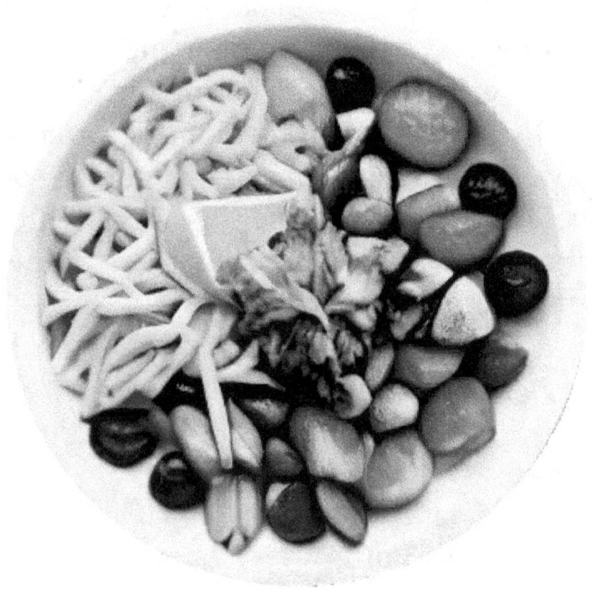

Chapter 6: Snacks and Desserts That Support Hormone Balance

Snacks and desserts play a crucial role in maintaining a balanced diet and supporting hormone health. The recipes in this chapter are designed to provide sustained energy and satisfy your sweet cravings while promoting overall well-being. Each recipe is crafted with nutrient-dense ingredients that are known to support hormone balance.

Recipe 57. Almond Butter Energy Bites

Ingredients:
- 1 cup rolled oats
- 1/2 cup almond butter
- 1/4 cup honey or maple syrup
- 1/4 cup ground flaxseed
- 1/4 cup dark chocolate chips
- 1 tsp vanilla extract

Method:
1. In a mixing bowl, combine rolled oats, almond butter, honey or maple syrup, ground flaxseed, dark chocolate chips, and vanilla extract.

2. Mix until well combined.
3. Roll the mixture into small balls, about 1 inch in diameter.
4. Place the energy bites on a baking sheet lined with parchment paper.
5. Refrigerate for at least 30 minutes before serving.

Preparation Time: 15 minutes
Nutritional Information:
- Calories: 150 kcal (per bite)
- Protein: 4g
- Carbohydrates: 18g
- Fat: 8g
- Fiber: 3g

Recipe 58. Spicy Roasted Chickpeas

Ingredients:
- 1 can (15 oz) chickpeas, drained and rinsed
- 1 tbsp olive oil
- 1 tsp paprika
- 1/2 tsp cayenne pepper
- 1/2 tsp garlic powder
- Salt and pepper to taste

Method:
1. Preheat the oven to 400°F (200°C).
2. Pat chickpeas dry with a paper towel.
3. In a bowl, toss chickpeas with olive oil, paprika, cayenne pepper, garlic powder, salt, and pepper.
4. Spread chickpeas in a single layer on a baking sheet.
5. Roast for 25-30 minutes until crispy, shaking the pan halfway through.
6. Let cool slightly before serving.

Preparation Time: 35 minutes
Nutritional Information:
- Calories: 180 kcal
- Protein: 8g
- Carbohydrates: 28g
- Fat: 5g
- Fiber: 6g

Recipe 59. Veggie Sticks with Hummus

Ingredients:
- 1 cup baby carrots
- 1 cup cucumber sticks
- 1 cup bell pepper strips
- 1/2 cup hummus

Method:
1. Arrange baby carrots, cucumber sticks, and bell pepper strips on a serving plate.
2. Serve with hummus for dipping.

Preparation Time: 5 minutes
Nutritional Information:
- Calories: 150 kcal
- Protein: 4g
- Carbohydrates: 20g
- Fat: 8g
- Fiber: 6g

Greek Yogurt with Honey and Nuts

Ingredients:
- 1 cup Greek yogurt
- 1 tbsp honey
- 2 tbsp mixed nuts (almonds, walnuts, pecans)

Method:
1. In a serving bowl, top Greek yogurt with honey and mixed nuts.
2. Serve immediately.

Preparation Time: 5 minutes
Nutritional Information:
- Calories: 200 kcal
- Protein: 12g
- Carbohydrates: 20g
- Fat: 9g
- Fiber: 2g

Recipe 60. Baked Kale Chips

Ingredients:
- 1 bunch kale, washed and torn into bite-sized pieces
- 1 tbsp olive oil
- 1/2 tsp salt

Method:
1. Preheat the oven to 350°F (175°C).
2. In a bowl, toss kale pieces with olive oil and salt.
3. Spread kale in a single layer on a baking sheet.
4. Bake for 10-15 minutes until crispy, turning once halfway through.
5. Let cool before serving.

Preparation Time: 20 minutes
Nutritional Information:
- Calories: 70 kcal
- Protein: 2g
- Carbohydrates: 7g
- Fat: 4g
- Fiber: 2g

Recipe 61. Apple Slices with Almond Butter

Ingredients:
- 1 apple, sliced
- 2 tbsp almond butter

Method:
1. Arrange apple slices on a plate.
2. Serve with almond butter for dipping.

Preparation Time: 5 minutes
Nutritional Information:
- Calories: 200 kcal
- Protein: 4g
- Carbohydrates: 28g
- Fat: 9g
- Fiber: 5g

 Edamame with Sea Salt

Ingredients:
- 1 cup edamame (fresh or frozen)
- 1/2 tsp sea salt

Method:
1. Cook edamame according to package instructions.
2. Sprinkle it with sea salt.

3. Serve warm.

Preparation Time: 10 minutes
Nutritional Information:
- Calories: 120 kcal
- Protein: 11g
- Carbohydrates: 9g
- Fat: 5g
- Fiber: 4g

Recipe 62. Mini Stuffed Mushrooms

Ingredients:
- 12 button mushrooms, stems removed
- 1/4 cup cream cheese
- 1/4 cup grated Parmesan cheese
- 1 clove garlic, minced
- 2 tbsp chopped fresh parsley
- Salt and pepper to taste

Method:
1. Preheat the oven to 375°F (190°C).
2. In a bowl, combine cream cheese, Parmesan cheese, minced garlic, fresh parsley, salt, and pepper.
3. Stuffed mushroom caps with the cheese mixture.
4. Place stuffed mushrooms on a baking sheet.
5. Bake for 15-20 minutes until mushrooms are tender and the filling is golden.
6. Serve warm.

Preparation Time: 30 minutes
Nutritional Information:
- Calories: 150 kcal (per 3 mushrooms)
- Protein: 6g
- Carbohydrates: 6g
- Fat: 12g

- Fiber: 2g
Recipe 63. Cucumber and Smoked Salmon Bites

Ingredients:
- 1 cucumber, sliced
- 4 oz smoked salmon
- 2 tbsp cream cheese
- 1 tbsp fresh dill, chopped

Method:
1. Spread a small amount of cream cheese on each cucumber slice.
2. Top with a piece of smoked salmon.
3. Garnish with fresh dill.
4. Serve immediately.

Preparation Time: 10 minutes
Nutritional Information:
- Calories: 100 kcal (per 6 bites)
- Protein: 6g
- Carbohydrates: 5g
- Fat: 6g
- Fiber: 1g

Recipe 64. Guacamole with Veggie Chips

Ingredients:
- 2 ripe avocados, mashed
- 1/4 cup red onion, finely chopped
- 1 small tomato, diced
- 1 clove garlic, minced
- Juice of 1 lime
- Salt and pepper to taste
- Veggie chips for serving

Method:
1. In a bowl, combine mashed avocados, red onion, tomato, minced garlic, and lime juice.
2. Season with salt and pepper.
3. Serve guacamole with veggie chips.

Preparation Time: 15 minutes
Nutritional Information:
- Calories: 200 kcal (per serving)
- Protein: 3g
- Carbohydrates: 20g
- Fat: 15g
- Fiber: 8g

Recipe 65. Shrimp Cocktail

Ingredients:
- 12 large shrimp, cooked and peeled
- 1/2 cup cocktail sauce
- Lemon wedges for serving

Method:
1. Arrange cooked shrimp on a serving plate.
2. Serve with cocktail sauce and lemon wedges.

Preparation Time: 10 minutes
Nutritional Information:
- Calories: 120 kcal (per 6 shrimp)
- Protein: 20g
- Carbohydrates: 10g
- Fat: 1g
- Fiber: 1g

Recipe 66. Stuffed Cherry Tomatoes

Ingredients:
- 12 cherry tomatoes
- 1/4 cup goat cheese
- 1 tbsp fresh basil, chopped
- Salt and pepper to taste

Method:
1. Slice the tops off the cherry tomatoes and scoop out the seeds.
2. In a bowl, mix goat cheese with fresh basil, salt, and pepper.
3. Stuff each cherry tomato with the goat cheese mixture.
4. Serve stuffed cherry tomatoes chilled.

Preparation Time: 15 minutes
Nutritional Information:
- Calories: 80 kcal (per 4 tomatoes)
- Protein: 3g
- Carbohydrates: 5g
- Fat: 5g
- Fiber: 1g

Recipe 67. Roasted Red Pepper Hummus with Veggies

Ingredients:
- 1 can (15 oz) chickpeas, drained and rinsed
- 1/4 cup roasted red peppers
- 2 tbsp tahini
- 1 clove garlic
- Juice of 1 lemon
- 2 tbsp olive oil
- Salt and pepper to taste
- Assorted fresh vegetables for dipping

Method:
1. In a food processor, combine chickpeas, roasted red peppers, tahini, garlic, lemon juice, and olive oil.
2. Blend until smooth, adding water if needed to reach desired consistency.
3. Season with salt and pepper.
4. Serve roasted red

pepper hummus with fresh vegetables.

Preparation Time: 15 minutes
Nutritional Information:
- Calories: 100 kcal (per 2 tbsp hummus)
- Protein: 4g

- Carbohydrates: 10g
- Fat: 5g
- Fiber: 3g

Recipe 68. Dark Chocolate Almond Bark

Ingredients:
- 8 oz dark chocolate, chopped
- 1/2 cup almonds, chopped

Method:
1. Melt dark chocolate in a microwave-safe bowl in 30-second intervals, stirring between each, until smooth.
2. Stir in chopped almonds.
3. Spread chocolate-almond mixture on a baking sheet lined with parchment paper.
4. Refrigerate until set, about 1 hour.
5. Break into pieces and serve.

Preparation Time: 10 minutes (plus 1 hour refrigeration)
Nutritional Information:
- Calories: 180 kcal (per piece)
- Protein: 3g
- Carbohydrates: 15g
- Fat: 12g
- Fiber: 4g

Recipe 69. Coconut Macaroons

Ingredients:
- 2 cups shredded coconut
- 2/3 cup sweetened condensed milk
- 1 tsp vanilla extract

Method:
1. Preheat the oven to 325°F (165°C).
2. In a bowl, mix shredded coconut, sweetened condensed milk, and vanilla extract.
3. Drop spoonfuls of the mixture onto a baking sheet lined with parchment paper.
4. Bake for 15-20 minutes until golden brown.
5. Let cool before serving.

Preparation Time: 25 minutes
Nutritional Information:
- Calories: 100 kcal (per macaroon)
- Protein: 1g
- Carbohydrates: 12g
- Fat: 5g
- Fiber: 2g

Recipe 70. Fresh Fruit Tart

Ingredients:
- 1 pre-made pie crust
- 1 cup Greek yogurt
- 2 tbsp honey
- 1 cup mixed fresh fruit (strawberries, blueberries, kiwi, etc.)

Method:
1. Preheat the oven to 375°F (190°C).
2. Bake premade pie crust according to package instructions. Let cool.
3. In a bowl, mix Greek yogurt and honey.
4. Spread yogurt mixture in the cooled pie crust.
5. Top with mixed fresh fruit.
6. Serve fresh fruit tart chilled.

Preparation Time: 30 minutes
Nutritional Information:
- Calories: 200 kcal (per slice)
- Protein: 6g
- Carbohydrates: 30g
- Fat: 8g
- Fiber: 3g

Recipe 71. Mango Sorbet

Ingredients:
- 2 ripe mangoes, peeled and diced
- 1/4 cup honey or agave nectar
- 1/2 cup water
- Juice of 1 lime

Method:
1. In a blender, combine diced mangoes, honey or agave nectar, water, and lime juice.
2. Blend until smooth.
3. Pour the mixture into an ice cream maker and churn according to the manufacturer's instructions.
4. Serve mango sorbet immediately or freeze until firm.

Preparation Time: 20 minutes (plus churning time)
Nutritional Information:
- Calories: 120 kcal (per serving)
- Protein: 1g
- Carbohydrates: 30g
- Fat: 0g
- Fiber: 2g

Recipe 72. Berry Compote with Greek Yogurt

Ingredients:
- 1 cup mixed berries (strawberries, blueberries, raspberries)
- 2 tbsp honey
- 1 cup Greek yogurt

Method:
1. In a saucepan, combine mixed berries and honey. Cook over medium heat until berries break down and form a compote, about 10 minutes.
2. In a serving bowl, layer Greek yogurt and berry compote.
3. Serve berry compote with Greek yogurt warm or chilled.

Preparation Time: 15 minutes
Nutritional Information:
- Calories: 180 kcal (per serving)
- Protein: 10g
- Carbohydrates: 30g
- Fat: 4g
- Fiber: 4g

Recipe 73. Almond Flour Brownies

Ingredients:
- 1 cup almond flour
- 1/2 cup cocoa powder
- 1/2 tsp baking powder
- 1/4 tsp salt
- 1/2 cup coconut sugar
- 1/4 cup coconut oil, melted
- 2 eggs
- 1 tsp vanilla extract

Method:
1. Preheat the oven to 350°F (175°C).
2. In a bowl, combine almond flour, cocoa powder, baking powder, and salt.
3. In a separate bowl, mix coconut sugar, melted coconut oil, eggs, and vanilla extract.
4. Combine wet and dry ingredients, mixing until smooth.
5. Pour batter into a greased baking pan.
6. Bake for 20-25 minutes until a toothpick inserted into the center comes out clean.
7. Let cool before cutting into squares.

Preparation Time: 30 minutes
Nutritional Information:

- Calories: 150 kcal (per brownie)
- Protein: 4g
- Carbohydrates: 15g
- Fat: 9g
- Fiber: 3g

Recipe 74. Lemon Poppy Seed Muffins

Ingredients:
- 1 cup almond flour
- 1/4 cup coconut flour
- 1/2 tsp baking soda
- 1/4 tsp salt
- 3 eggs
- 1/4 cup honey
- 1/4 cup coconut oil, melted
- Juice and zest of 1 lemon
- 1 tbsp poppy seeds

Method:
1. Preheat the oven to 350°F (175°C).
2. In a bowl, combine almond flour, coconut flour, baking soda, and salt.
3. In a separate bowl, mix eggs, honey, melted coconut oil, lemon juice, and zest.
4. Combine wet and dry ingredients, mixing until smooth.
5. Stir in poppy seeds.
6. Divide batter into a greased muffin tin.
7. Bake for 20-25 minutes until a toothpick inserted into the center comes out clean.
8. Let cool before serving.

Preparation Time: 30 minutes

Nutritional Information:
- Calories: 120 kcal (per muffin)
- Protein: 4g
- Carbohydrates: 10g
- Fat: 8g
- Fiber: 2g

Recipe 75. Flourless Chocolate Cake
Ingredients:
- 1 cup dark chocolate chips
- 1/2 cup butter
- 3/4 cup sugar
- 3 eggs
- 1/2 cup cocoa powder

Method:
1. Preheat the oven to 375°F (190°C).
2. Melt dark chocolate chips and butter together in a microwave-safe bowl, stirring until smooth.
3. Stir in sugar, then add eggs one at a time, mixing well after each addition.
4. Sift in cocoa powder and mix until smooth.
5. Pour batter into a greased cake pan.
6. Bake for 20-25 minutes until a toothpick inserted into the center comes out with a few moist crumbs.
7. Let cool before serving.

Preparation Time: 35 minutes
Nutritional Information:
- Calories: 220 kcal (per slice)
- Protein: 4g
- Carbohydrates: 25g
- Fat: 12g
- Fiber: 4g

Recipe 76. Almond Butter Cookies

Ingredients:
- 1 cup almond butter
- 1/2 cup coconut sugar
- 1 egg
- 1 tsp vanilla extract
- 1/2 tsp baking soda

Method:
1. Preheat the oven to 350°F (175°C).
2. In a bowl, mix almond butter, coconut sugar, egg, vanilla extract, and baking soda until well combined.
3. Drop spoonfuls of dough onto a baking sheet lined with parchment paper.
4. Bake for 10-12 minutes until the edges are golden.
5. Let cool before serving.

Preparation Time: 20 minutes
Nutritional Information:
- Calories: 130 kcal (per cookie)
- Protein: 4g
- Carbohydrates: 12g
- Fat: 8g
- Fiber: 2g

Recipe 77. Pumpkin Spice Muffins

Ingredients:
- 1 cup almond flour
- 1/4 cup coconut flour
- 1/2 tsp baking soda
- 1/4 tsp salt
- 1/2 cup pumpkin puree
- 3 eggs
- 1/4 cup honey
- 1/4 cup coconut oil, melted
- 1 tsp pumpkin pie spice

Method:
1. Preheat the oven to 350°F (175°C).
2. In a bowl, combine almond flour, coconut flour, baking soda, and salt.
3. In a separate bowl, mix pumpkin puree, eggs, honey, melted coconut oil, and pumpkin pie spice.
4. Combine wet and dry ingredients, mixing until smooth.
5. Divide batter into a greased muffin tin.
6. Bake for 20-25 minutes until a toothpick inserted into the center comes out clean.
7. Let cool before serving.

Preparation Time: 30 minutes
Nutritional Information:
- Calories: 130 kcal (per muffin)
- Protein: 4g
- Carbohydrates: 10g
- Fat: 8g
- Fiber: 3g

Recipe 78. Carrot Cake Bites

Ingredients:
- 1 cup grated carrots
- 1 cup almond flour
- 1/2 cup shredded coconut
- 1/4 cup honey
- 1/4 cup almond butter
- 1 tsp vanilla extract
- 1/2 tsp ground cinnamon
- 1/4 tsp ground nutmeg
- 1/4 tsp salt

Method:
1. In a mixing bowl, combine grated carrots, almond flour, shredded coconut, honey, almond butter, vanilla extract, ground cinnamon, ground nutmeg, and salt.
2. Mix until well combined.
3. Roll the mixture into small balls, about 1 inch in diameter.
4. Place the carrot cake bites on a baking sheet lined with parchment paper.
5. Refrigerate for at least 30 minutes before serving.

Preparation Time: 15 minutes
Nutritional Information:

- Calories: 100 kcal (per bite)
- Protein: 2g
- Carbohydrates: 10g
- Fat: 6g
- Fiber: 2g

Recipe 79. Chocolate Avocado Mousse

Ingredients:
- 2 ripe avocados, pitted and peeled
- 1/4 cup cocoa powder
- 1/4 cup honey or maple syrup
- 1/4 cup almond milk
- 1 tsp vanilla extract
- Pinch of salt

Method:
1. In a food processor, combine avocados, cocoa powder, honey or maple syrup, almond milk, vanilla extract, and a pinch of salt.
2. Blend until smooth and creamy.
3. Spoon the mousse into serving bowls and refrigerate for at least 30 minutes before serving.

Preparation Time: 10 minutes
Nutritional Information:
- Calories: 180 kcal (per serving)
- Protein: 2g
- Carbohydrates: 20g
- Fat: 12g
- Fiber: 6g

Recipe 80. Blueberry Almond Crumble

Ingredients:
- 2 cups fresh blueberries
- 1 tbsp honey
- 1/2 cup almond flour
- 1/4 cup rolled oats
- 1/4 cup chopped almonds
- 2 tbsp coconut oil, melted
- 1/2 tsp ground cinnamon
- Pinch of salt

Method:
1. Preheat the oven to 350°F (175°C).
2. In a bowl, toss blueberries with honey and spread in a baking dish.
3. In another bowl, combine almond flour, rolled oats, chopped almonds, melted coconut oil, ground cinnamon, and a pinch of salt.
4. Sprinkle the almond mixture over the blueberries.
5. Bake for 25-30 minutes until the topping is golden and the blueberries are bubbly.
6. Let cool slightly before serving.

Preparation Time: 35 minutes
Nutritional Information:
- Calories: 150 kcal (per serving)

- Protein: 3g
- Carbohydrates: 20g
- Fat: 8g
- Fiber: 4g

Tips for Maintaining Hormone Balance

Maintaining hormone balance involves more than just incorporating hormone-supportive snacks and desserts into your diet. Here are some additional tips to support overall hormonal health:

1. Prioritize Whole Foods: Focus on eating whole, unprocessed foods that provide essential nutrients and healthy fats.
2. Manage Stress: High stress levels can disrupt hormone balance. Practice stress management techniques such as mindfulness, yoga, and deep breathing exercises.
3. Stay Hydrated: Proper hydration is crucial for overall health and can aid in maintaining hormone balance.

4. Exercise Regularly: Regular physical activity helps regulate hormones and improves overall well-being.

5. Get Adequate Sleep: Quality sleep is vital for hormone production and regulation. Aim for 7-9 hours of sleep per night.

6. Avoid Toxins: Limit exposure to environmental toxins that can disrupt hormonal balance. Opt for natural and organic products when possible.

7. Monitor Caffeine and Alcohol Intake: Excessive caffeine and alcohol can negatively impact hormone levels. Consume these in moderation.

8. Support Gut Health: A healthy gut is essential for hormone balance. Include probiotics and prebiotics in your diet to promote a healthy digestive system.

9. Consult with a Healthcare Provider: Regular check-ups with a healthcare provider can help monitor hormone levels and address any imbalances early on.

By integrating these hormone-supportive snacks and desserts into your diet, along with following these lifestyle tips, you can take proactive steps towards maintaining hormone balance and overall health. Enjoy these delicious recipes and take care of your body, mind, and spirit for a harmonious life.

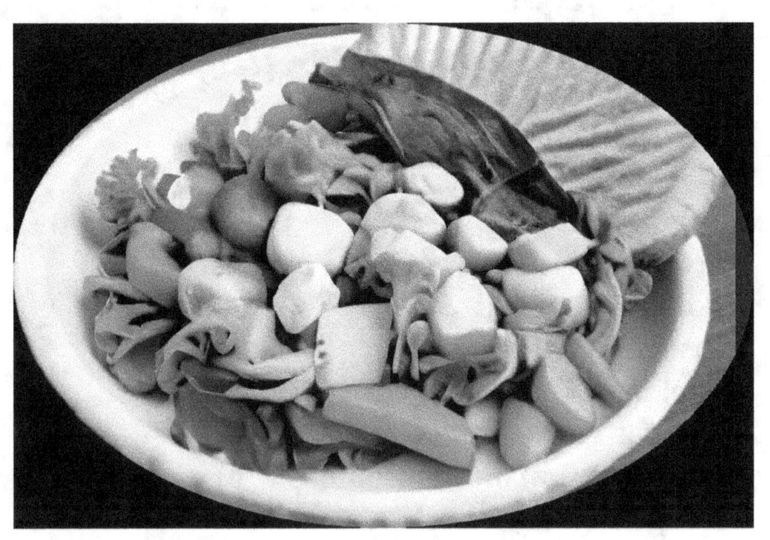

Chapter 7: Nourishing Soups and Stews

Recipe 81. Lentil and Vegetable Soup

Ingredients:
- 1 cup dried lentils, rinsed
- 1 onion, chopped
- 2 carrots, chopped
- 2 celery stalks, chopped
- 3 cloves garlic, minced
- 1 can (14.5 oz) diced tomatoes
- 6 cups vegetable broth
- 1 tsp dried thyme
- 1 tsp dried oregano
- 1 bay leaf
- Salt and pepper to taste
- 2 cups chopped spinach

Method:
1. In a large pot, sauté onion, carrots, and celery over medium heat until softened, about 5 minutes.
2. Add garlic and cook for another minute.

3. Add lentils, diced tomatoes, vegetable broth, thyme, oregano, and bay leaf. Bring to a boil.

4. Reduce heat and simmer for 25-30 minutes, until lentils are tender.

5. Stir in spinach and cook for an additional 5 minutes.

6. Season with salt and pepper to taste. Remove bay leaf before serving.

Cooking Time: 45 minutes
Nutritional Information:
- Calories: 200 kcal (per serving)
- Protein: 12g
- Carbohydrates: 35g
- Fat: 3g
- Fiber: 15g

Recipe 82. Chicken and Vegetable Soup

Ingredients:
- 1 lb boneless, skinless chicken breasts, diced
- 1 onion, chopped
- 2 carrots, sliced
- 2 celery stalks, sliced
- 3 cloves garlic, minced
- 1 zucchini, chopped
- 1 cup green beans, trimmed and cut
- 6 cups chicken broth
- 1 tsp dried thyme
- 1 tsp dried rosemary
- Salt and pepper to taste
- 2 tbsp olive oil

Method:
1. In a large pot, heat olive oil over medium heat. Add onion, carrots, and celery, and sauté until softened, about 5 minutes.
2. Add garlic and cook for another minute.
3. Add chicken and cook until browned, about 5 minutes.
4. Add zucchini, green beans, chicken broth, thyme, and rosemary. Bring to a boil.
5. Reduce heat and simmer for 20-25 minutes, until vegetables are tender and chicken is cooked through.

6. Season with salt and pepper to taste.

Cooking Time: 40 minutes
Nutritional Information:
- **Calories: 250 kcal (per serving)**
- **Protein: 25g**
- **Carbohydrates: 18g**
- **Fat: 10g**
- **Fiber: 6g**

Recipe 83. Sweet Potato and Kale Soup

Ingredients:
- 2 large sweet potatoes, peeled and cubed
- 1 onion, chopped
- 3 cloves garlic, minced
- 6 cups vegetable broth
- 1 tsp ground cumin
- 1 tsp smoked paprika
- 1/2 tsp ground cinnamon
- Salt and pepper to taste
- 4 cups chopped kale
- 2 tbsp olive oil

Method:
1. In a large pot, heat olive oil over medium heat. Add onion and sauté until softened, about 5 minutes.
2. Add garlic and cook for another minute.
3. Add sweet potatoes, vegetable broth, cumin, smoked paprika, and cinnamon. Bring to a boil.
4. Reduce heat and simmer for 20-25 minutes, until sweet potatoes are tender.
5. Add kale and cook for an additional 5 minutes.
6. Season with salt and pepper to taste.

Cooking Time: 35 minutes
Nutritional Information:

- Calories: 220 kcal (per serving)
- Protein: 5g
- Carbohydrates: 40g
- Fat: 6g
- Fiber: 8g

Recipe 84. Mushroom and Barley Soup

Ingredients:
- 1 cup pearl barley
- 1 lb mushrooms, sliced
- 1 onion, chopped
- 2 carrots, sliced
- 3 cloves garlic, minced
- 6 cups vegetable broth
- 1 tsp dried thyme
- 1 tsp dried rosemary
- Salt and pepper to taste
- 2 tbsp olive oil

Method:
1. In a large pot, heat olive oil over medium heat. Add onion and carrots, and sauté until softened, about 5 minutes.
2. Add garlic and mushrooms, and cook until mushrooms release their juices, about 5 minutes.
3. Add barley, vegetable broth, thyme, and rosemary. Bring to a boil.
4. Reduce heat and simmer for 45-50 minutes, until barley is tender.
5. Season with salt and pepper to taste.

Cooking Time: 60 minutes
Nutritional Information:

- Calories: 230 kcal (per serving)
- Protein: 7g
- Carbohydrates: 40g
- Fat: 5g
- Fiber: 8g

Recipe 85. Turkey and Spinach Stew

Ingredients:
- 1 lb ground turkey
- 1 onion, chopped
- 2 carrots, chopped
- 3 cloves garlic, minced
- 1 can (14.5 oz) diced tomatoes
- 4 cups chicken broth
- 1 tsp dried thyme
- 1 tsp dried oregano
- Salt and pepper to taste
- 4 cups spinach
- 2 tbsp olive oil

Method:
1. In a large pot, heat olive oil over medium heat. Add onion and carrots, and sauté until softened, about 5 minutes.
2. Add garlic and ground turkey, and cook until turkey is browned, about 5 minutes.
3. Add diced tomatoes, chicken broth, thyme, and oregano. Bring to a boil.
4. Reduce heat and simmer for 20-25 minutes, until vegetables are tender.
5. Stir in spinach and cook for an additional 5 minutes.
6. Season with salt and pepper to taste.

Cooking Time: 35 minutes
Nutritional Information:
- Calories: 250 kcal (per serving)
- Protein: 25g
- Carbohydrates: 20g
- Fat: 10g
- Fiber: 6g

Recipe 86. Spiced Butternut Squash Soup

Ingredients:
- 1 large butternut squash, peeled, seeded, and cubed
- 1 onion, chopped
- 3 cloves garlic, minced
- 6 cups vegetable broth
- 1 tsp ground cumin
- 1 tsp ground coriander
- 1/2 tsp ground cinnamon
- Salt and pepper to taste
- 2 tbsp olive oil

Method:
1. In a large pot, heat olive oil over medium heat. Add onion and sauté until softened, about 5 minutes.
2. Add garlic and cook for another minute.
3. Add butternut squash, vegetable broth, cumin, coriander, and cinnamon. Bring to a boil.
4. Reduce heat and simmer for 20-25 minutes, until squash is tender.
5. Puree the soup using an immersion blender or in batches in a regular blender until smooth.
6. Season with salt and pepper to taste.

Cooking Time: 35 minutes

Nutritional Information:
- Calories: 180 kcal (per serving)
- Protein: 3g
- Carbohydrates: 35g
- Fat: 6g
- Fiber: 7g

Chapter 8: Recipes for Healthy Digestion

Recipe 87. Fermented Carrot and Ginger Salad

Ingredients:
- 4 large carrots, grated
- 1 tbsp grated fresh ginger
- 1 tsp sea salt
- 1/2 cup water

Method:
1. In a bowl, mix grated carrots, ginger, and sea salt.
2. Pack the mixture tightly into a mason jar, leaving about an inch of space at the top.
3. Pour water over the mixture until it is completely submerged.
4. Cover the jar with a lid and let it sit at room temperature for 3-5 days to ferment.
5. Once fermented, store in the refrigerator and serve chilled.

Preparation Time: 10 minutes + 3-5 days fermentation
Nutritional Information:

- Calories: 50 kcal (per serving)
- Protein: 1g
- Carbohydrates: 10g
- Fat: 0g
- Fiber: 3g

Recipe 88. Probiotic-Rich Smoothie

Ingredients:
- 1 cup kefir or plain yogurt
- 1 banana
- 1/2 cup frozen berries
- 1 tbsp chia seeds
- 1 tbsp honey
- 1/2 tsp vanilla extract

Method:
1. In a blender, combine kefir or yogurt, banana, frozen berries, chia seeds, honey, and vanilla extract.
2. Blend until smooth.
3. Pour into a glass and serve immediately.

Preparation Time: 5 minutes
Nutritional Information:
- Calories: 200 kcal (per serving)
- Protein: 8g
- Carbohydrates: 35g
- Fat: 4g
- Fiber: 6g

Recipe 89. Gut-Healing Bone Broth

Ingredients:
- 2 lbs beef bones
- 2 carrots, chopped
- 2 celery stalks, chopped
- 1 onion, chopped
- 3 cloves garlic, smashed
- 1 tbsp apple cider vinegar
- 10 cups water
- 1 tsp sea salt
- 1 tsp black peppercorns
- 2 bay leaves

Method:

1. Place all ingredients in a large pot or slow cooker.
2. Bring to a boil, then reduce heat and simmer for 12-24 hours.
3. Strain the broth through a fine-mesh sieve and discard the solids.
4. Store the broth in the refrigerator for up to a week or freeze for later use.

Cooking Time: 12-24 hours
Nutritional Information:

- Calories: 50 kcal (per serving)
- Protein: 5g
- Carbohydrates: 2g
- Fat: 2g
- Fiber: 0g

Recipe 90. Yogurt and Berry Breakfast Bowl

Ingredients:
- 1 cup plain Greek yogurt
- 1/2 cup mixed berries
- 1 tbsp honey
- 1 tbsp chia seeds
- 1 tbsp sliced almonds

Method:
1. In a bowl, combine Greek yogurt and honey.
2. Top with mixed berries, chia seeds, and sliced almonds.
3. Serve immediately.

Preparation Time: 5 minutes
Nutritional Information:
- Calories: 200 kcal (per serving)
- Protein: 15g
- Carbohydrates: 25g
- Fat: 5g
- Fiber: 5g

Recipe 91. Fiber-Rich Chia Pudding

Ingredients:
- 1/4 cup chia seeds
- 1 cup almond milk
- 1 tbsp honey or maple syrup
- 1/2 tsp vanilla extract
- Fresh fruit for topping (optional)

Method:
1. In a bowl, combine chia seeds, almond milk, honey or maple syrup, and vanilla extract.
2. Stir well and let sit for 10 minutes, then stir again.
3. Cover and refrigerate for at least 2 hours or overnight.
4. Serve with fresh fruit if desired.

Preparation Time: 5 minutes + 2 hours refrigeration
Nutritional Information:
- Calories: 180 kcal (per serving)
- Protein: 5g
- Carbohydrates: 20g
- Fat: 9g
- Fiber: 12g

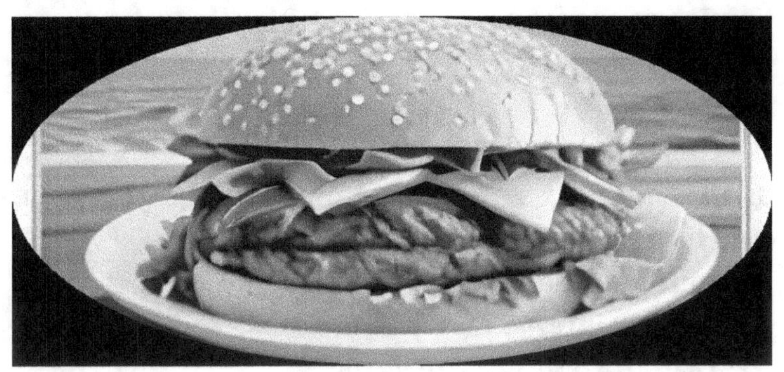

Chapter 9: Anti-Inflammatory Recipes for Vitality

Recipe 92. Turmeric and Ginger Tea

Ingredients:
- 1 tsp ground turmeric
- 1 tsp grated fresh ginger
- 1 tbsp honey
- Juice of 1 lemon
- 2 cups hot water

Method:
1. In a teapot, combine turmeric, ginger, honey, and lemon juice.
2. Pour hot water over the mixture and let steep for 5-10 minutes.
3. Strain into mugs and serve.

Preparation Time: 10 minutes
Nutritional Information:
- Calories: 40 kcal (per serving)
- Protein: 0g
- Carbohydrates: 10g
- Fat: 0g
- Fiber: 1g

Recipe 93. Anti-Inflammatory Smoothie

Ingredients:
- 1 cup almond milk
- 1/2 cup frozen pineapple
- 1/2 cup frozen mango
- 1 banana
- 1 tsp ground turmeric
- 1 tsp grated fresh ginger
- 1 tbsp honey
- 1 tbsp chia seeds

Method:
1. In a blender, combine almond milk, pineapple, mango, banana, turmeric, ginger, honey, and chia seeds.
2. Blend until smooth.
3. Pour into a glass and serve immediately.

Preparation Time: 5 minutes
Nutritional Information:
- Calories: 250 kcal (per serving)
- Protein: 3g
- Carbohydrates: 55g
- Fat: 4g
- Fiber: 8g

Recipe 94. Grilled Salmon with Avocado Salsa

Ingredients:
- 4 salmon filets
- 2 avocados, diced
- 1 tomato, diced
- 1/4 cup red onion, diced
- Juice of 1 lime
- 2 tbsp chopped cilantro
- Salt and pepper to taste
- 2 tbsp olive oil

Method:
1. Preheat the grill to medium-high heat.
2. Season salmon filets with salt and pepper and brush with olive oil.
3. Grill salmon for 4-5 minutes per side, until cooked through.
4. In a bowl, combine diced avocados, tomato, red onion, lime juice, and cilantro. Season with salt and pepper to taste.
5. Serve grilled salmon topped with avocado salsa.

Cooking Time: 15 minutes
Nutritional Information:
- Calories: 350 kcal (per serving)
- Protein: 30g
- Carbohydrates: 15g
- Fat: 20g

- Fiber: 7g

Recipe 95. Spinach and Berry Salad

Ingredients:
- 4 cups fresh spinach
- 1 cup mixed berries (strawberries, blueberries, raspberries)
- 1/4 cup crumbled feta cheese
- 1/4 cup chopped walnuts
- 2 tbsp balsamic vinaigrette

Method:
1. In a large bowl, combine spinach, mixed berries, feta cheese, and walnuts.
2. Drizzle with balsamic vinaigrette and toss to combine.
3. Serve immediately.

Preparation Time: 10 minutes
Nutritional Information:
- Calories: 200 kcal (per serving)
- Protein: 5g
- Carbohydrates: 20g
- Fat: 12g
- Fiber: 5g

Recipe 96. Roasted Vegetables with Turmeric

Ingredients:
- 2 cups broccoli florets
- 2 cups cauliflower florets
- 2 carrots, sliced
- 1 red bell pepper, chopped
- 2 tbsp olive oil
- 1 tsp ground turmeric
- Salt and pepper to taste

Method:
1. Preheat the oven to 400°F (200°C).
2. In a large bowl, toss vegetables with olive oil, turmeric, salt, and pepper.
3. Spread the vegetables on a baking sheet in a single layer.
4. Roast for 25-30 minutes, until tender and lightly browned.
5. Serve immediately.

Cooking Time: 35 minutes
Nutritional Information:
- Calories: 150 kcal (per serving)
- Protein: 4g
- Carbohydrates: 18g
- Fat: 8g
- Fiber: 6g

Recipe 97. Chia and Flaxseed Crackers

Ingredients:
- 1/2 cup chia seeds
- 1/2 cup ground flaxseeds
- 1/2 cup water
- 1/2 tsp salt
- 1/2 tsp garlic powder
- 1/2 tsp onion powder

Method:
1. Preheat the oven to 325°F (165°C).
2. In a bowl, combine chia seeds, ground flaxseeds, water, salt, garlic powder, and onion powder.
3. Mix well and let sit for 10 minutes to thicken.
4. Spread the mixture evenly on a baking sheet lined with parchment paper.
5. Bake for 30-35 minutes, until crisp.
6. Let cool and break into pieces.

Cooking Time: 45 minutes
Nutritional Information:
- Calories: 100 kcal (per serving)
- Protein: 3g
- Carbohydrates: 8g
- Fat: 7g

- Fiber: 7g

<u>Final Thoughts</u>

Eating for vitality and energy doesn't have to be complicated. With the right recipes and a focus on nutrient-dense foods, you can support your body's natural processes and enjoy improved well-being.

These nourishing soups, stews, digestive-friendly dishes, and anti-inflammatory recipes are designed to provide you with the nutrients you need to thrive.

Remember, a balanced diet and healthy lifestyle go hand-in-hand in promoting long-term health and vitality.

Enjoy these recipes as part of your journey towards a healthier, more vibrant life.

Chapter 10: Creating a Meal Plan That Works for You

Weekly Meal Plan Template

Creating a weekly meal plan is an essential step in ensuring you stick to the Galveston Diet and make the most out of your healthy eating journey. A well-organized meal plan can help you save time, reduce stress, and ensure you have balanced and nutritious meals throughout the week.

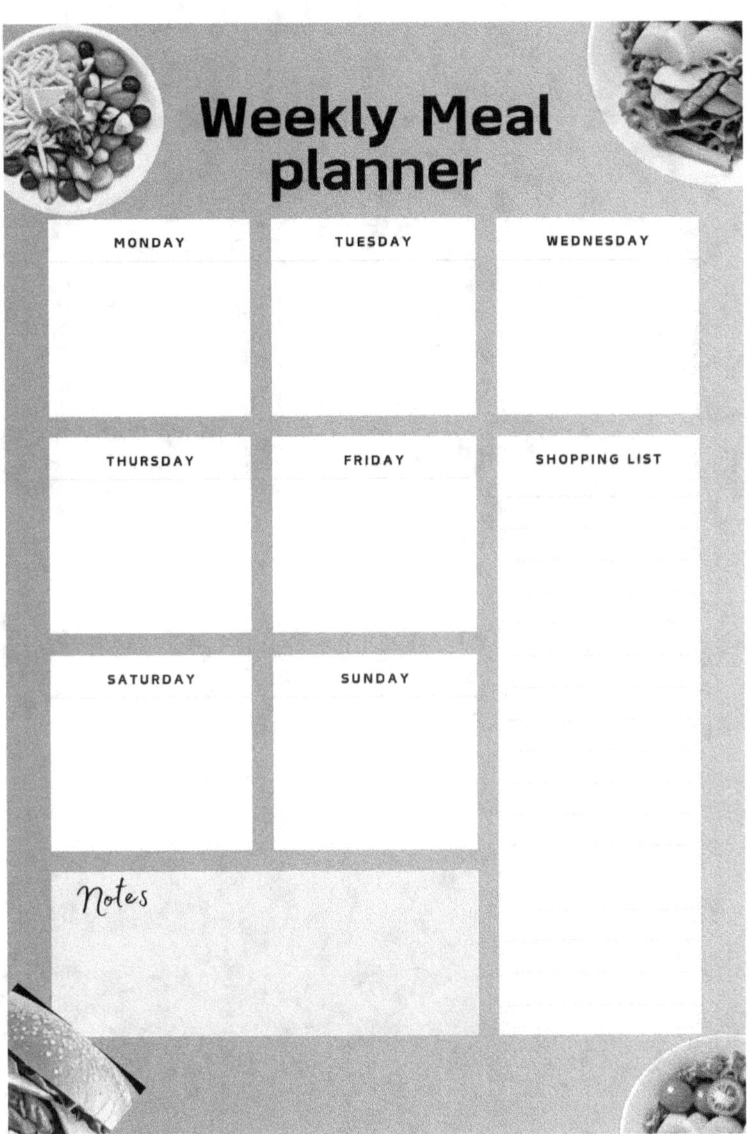

Weekly Meal planner
MONDAY
TUESDAY
WEDNESDAY
THURSDAY
FRIDAY
SHOPPING LIST
SATURDAY
SUNDAY
Notes

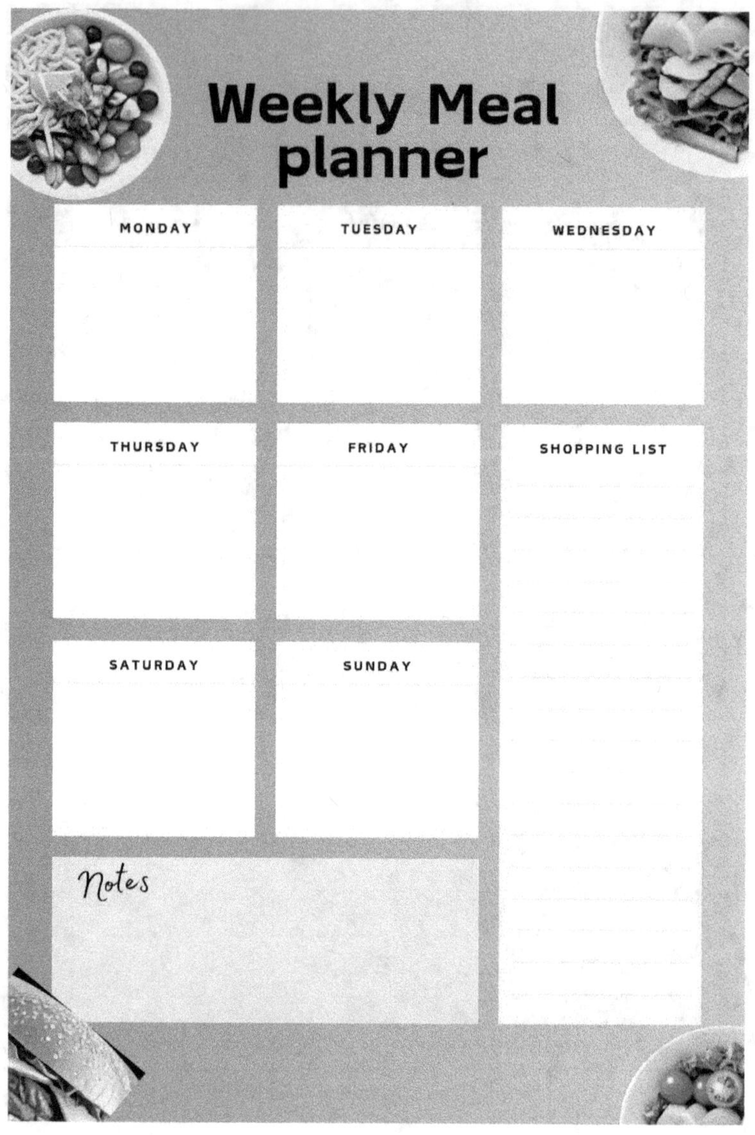
Weekly Meal planner
MONDAY
TUESDAY
WEDNESDAY
THURSDAY
FRIDAY
SHOPPING LIST
SATURDAY
SUNDAY
Notes

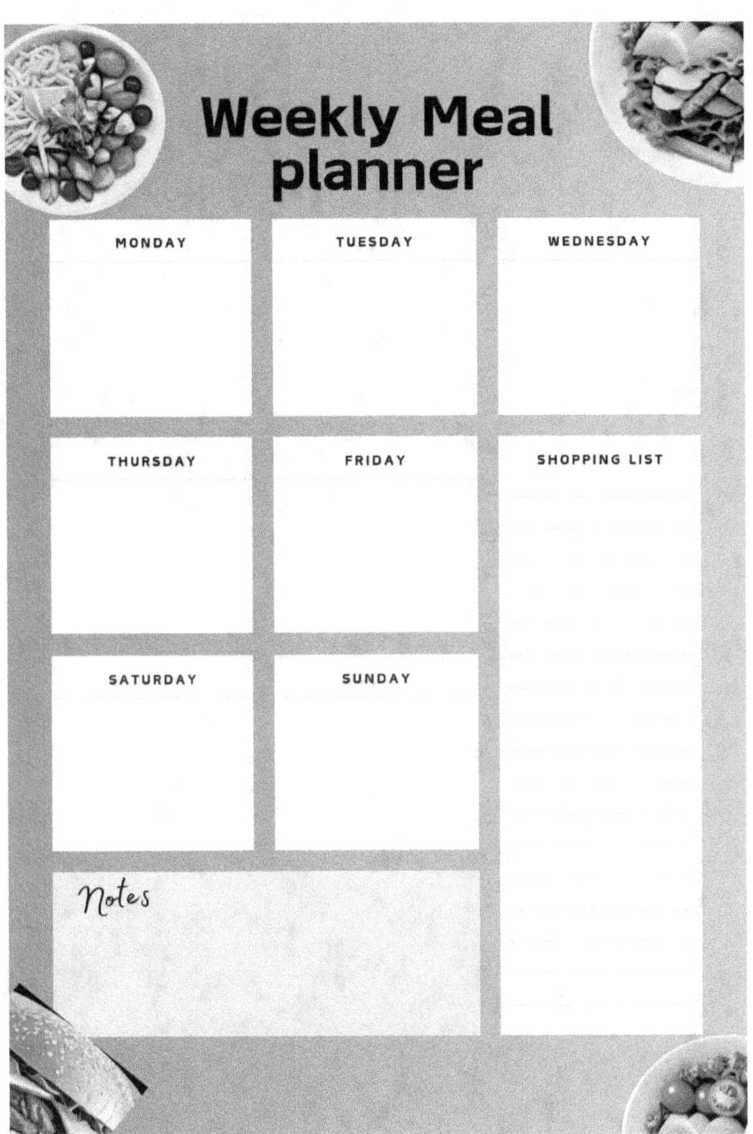

Weekly Meal planner
MONDAY
TUESDAY
WEDNESDAY
THURSDAY
FRIDAY
SHOPPING LIST
SATURDAY
SUNDAY
Notes

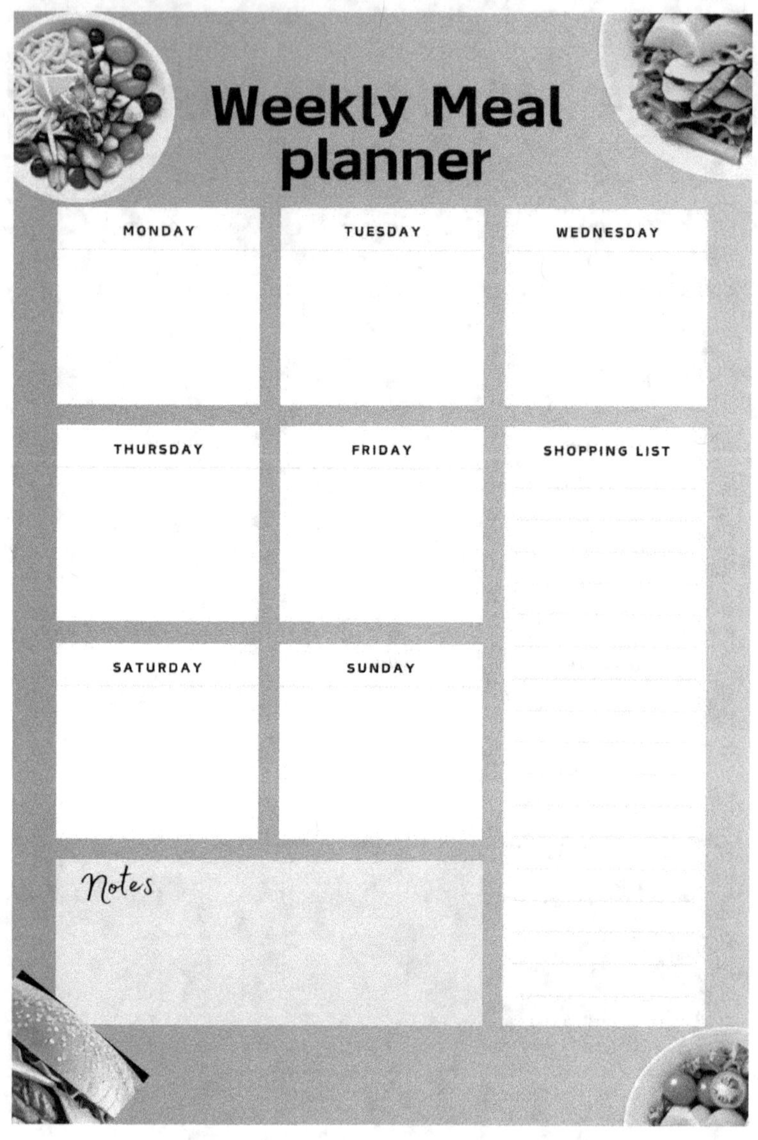

Weekly Meal planner
MONDAY
TUESDAY
WEDNESDAY
THURSDAY
FRIDAY
SHOPPING LIST
SATURDAY
SUNDAY
Notes

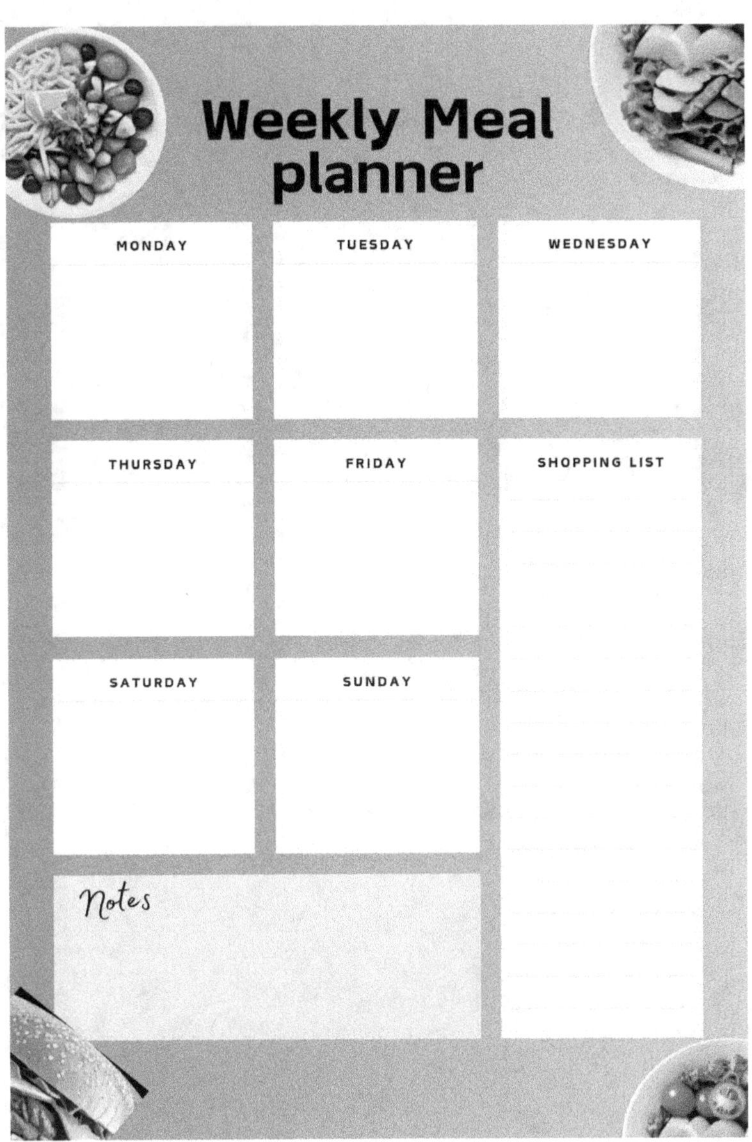

Weekly Meal planner
MONDAY
TUESDAY
WEDNESDAY
THURSDAY
FRIDAY
SHOPPING LIST
SATURDAY
SUNDAY
Notes

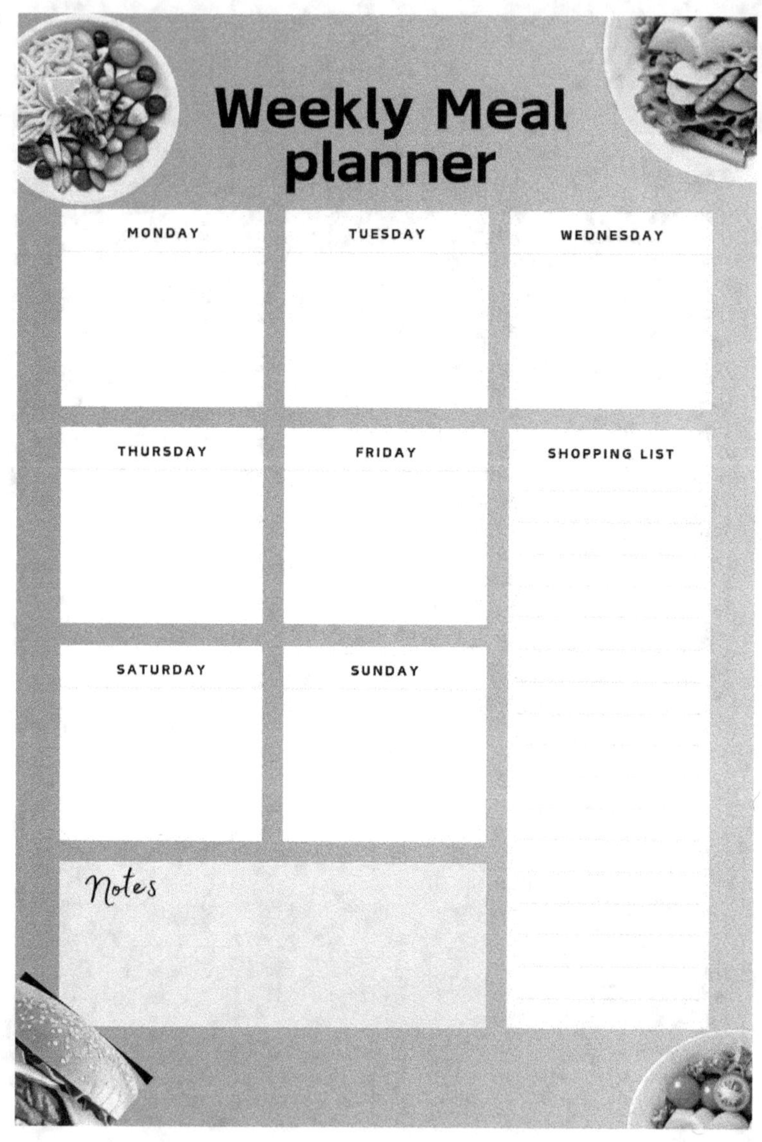

181

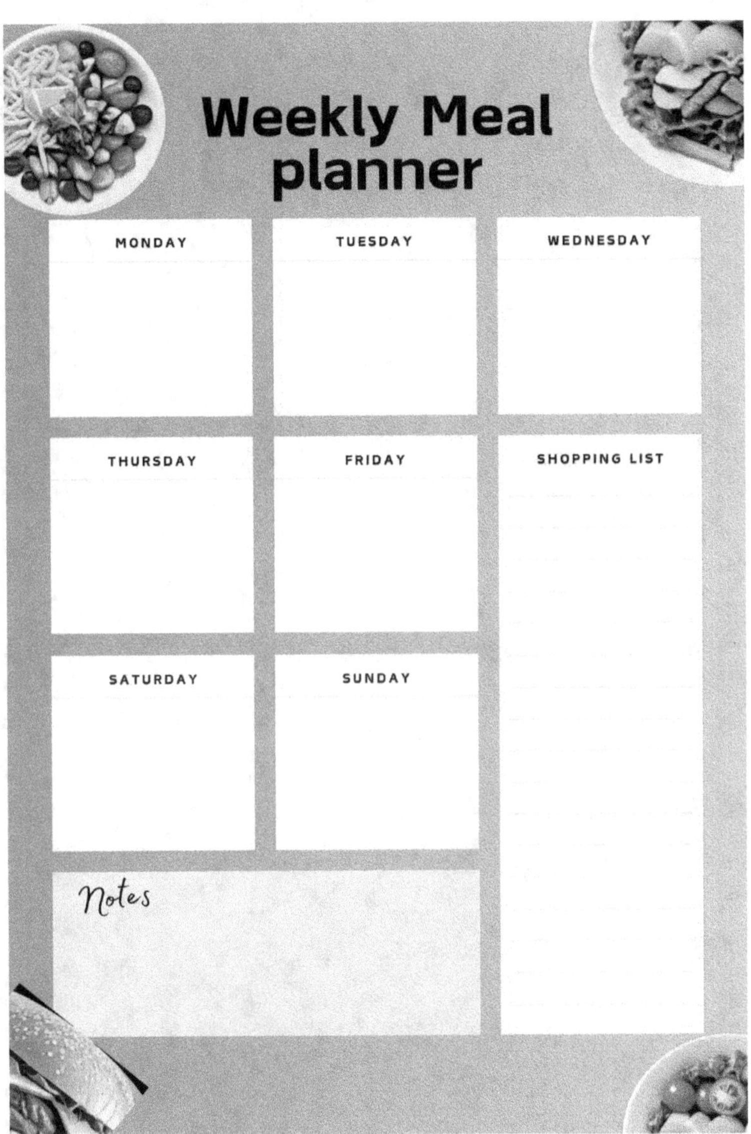

Weekly Meal planner
MONDAY
TUESDAY
WEDNESDAY
THURSDAY
FRIDAY
SHOPPING LIST
SATURDAY
SUNDAY
Notes

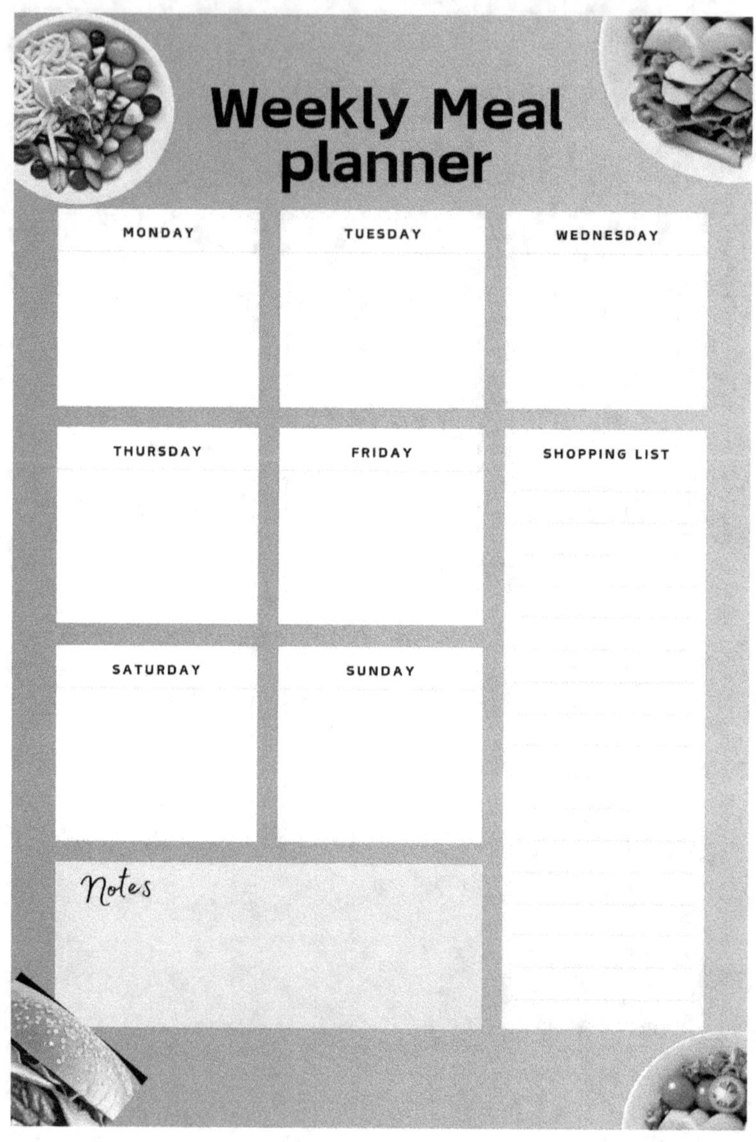

Weekly Meal planner
MONDAY
TUESDAY
WEDNESDAY
THURSDAY
FRIDAY
SHOPPING LIST
SATURDAY
SUNDAY
Notes

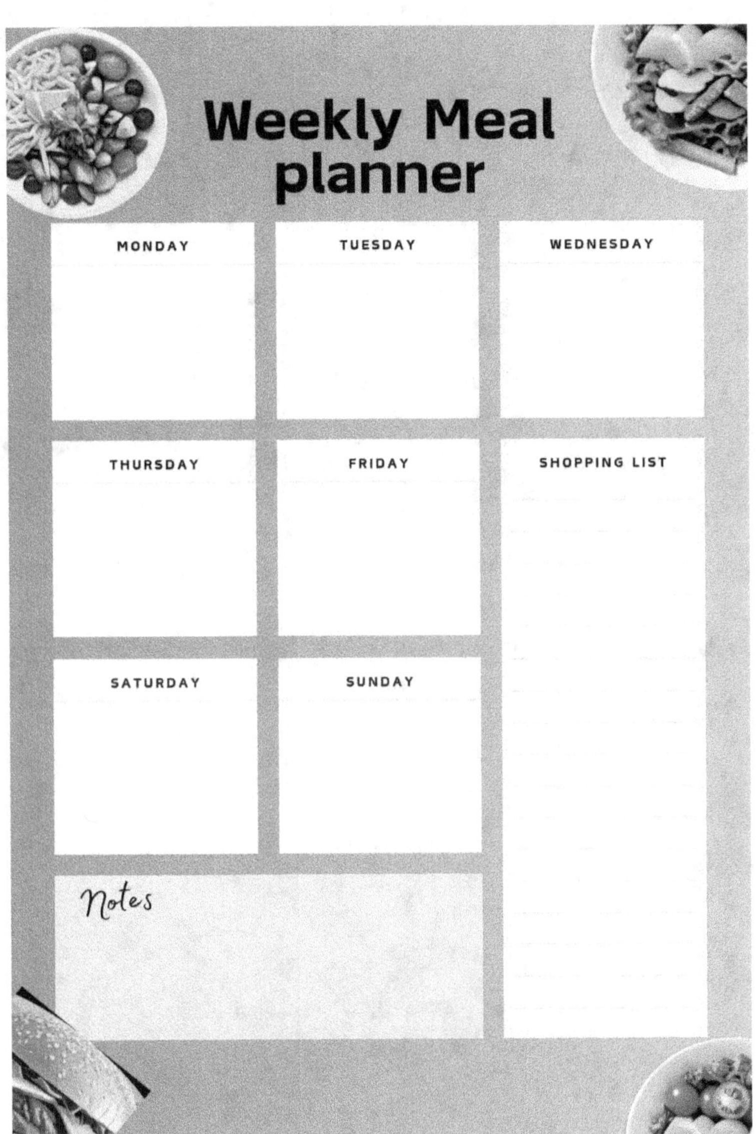

Weekly Meal planner
MONDAY
TUESDAY
WEDNESDAY
THURSDAY
FRIDAY
SHOPPING LIST
SATURDAY
SUNDAY
Notes

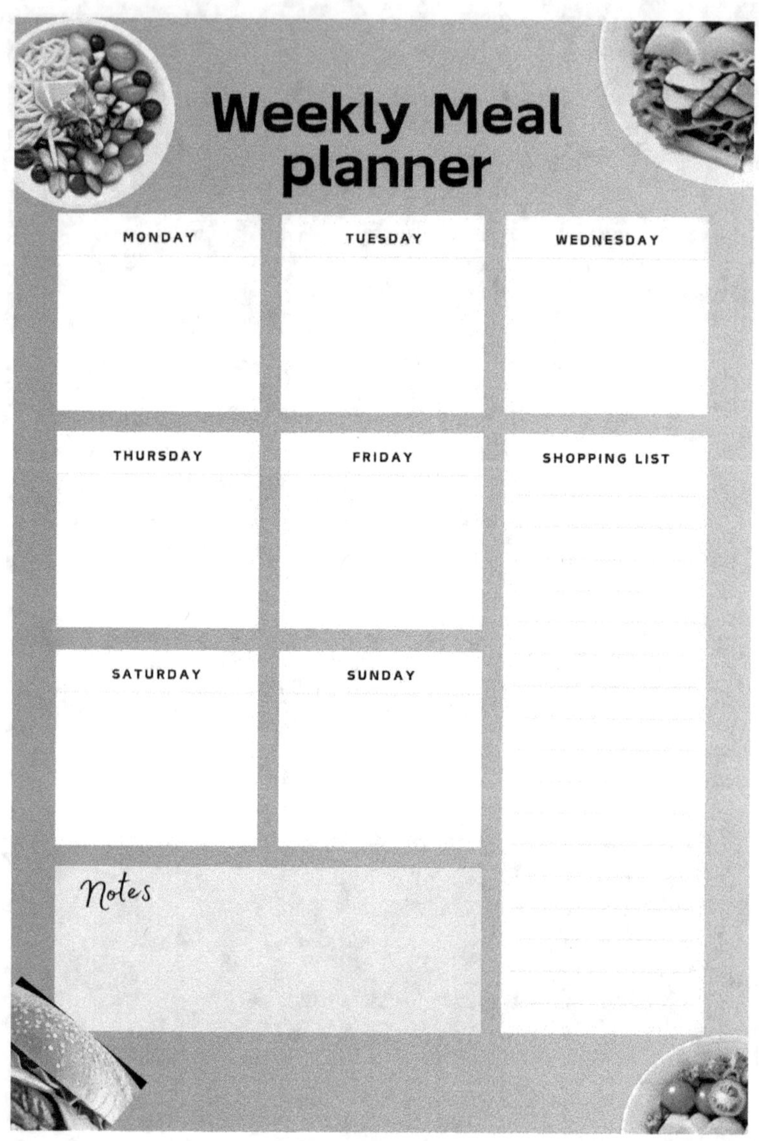

Weekly Meal planner
MONDAY
TUESDAY
WEDNESDAY
THURSDAY
FRIDAY
SHOPPING LIST
SATURDAY
SUNDAY
Notes

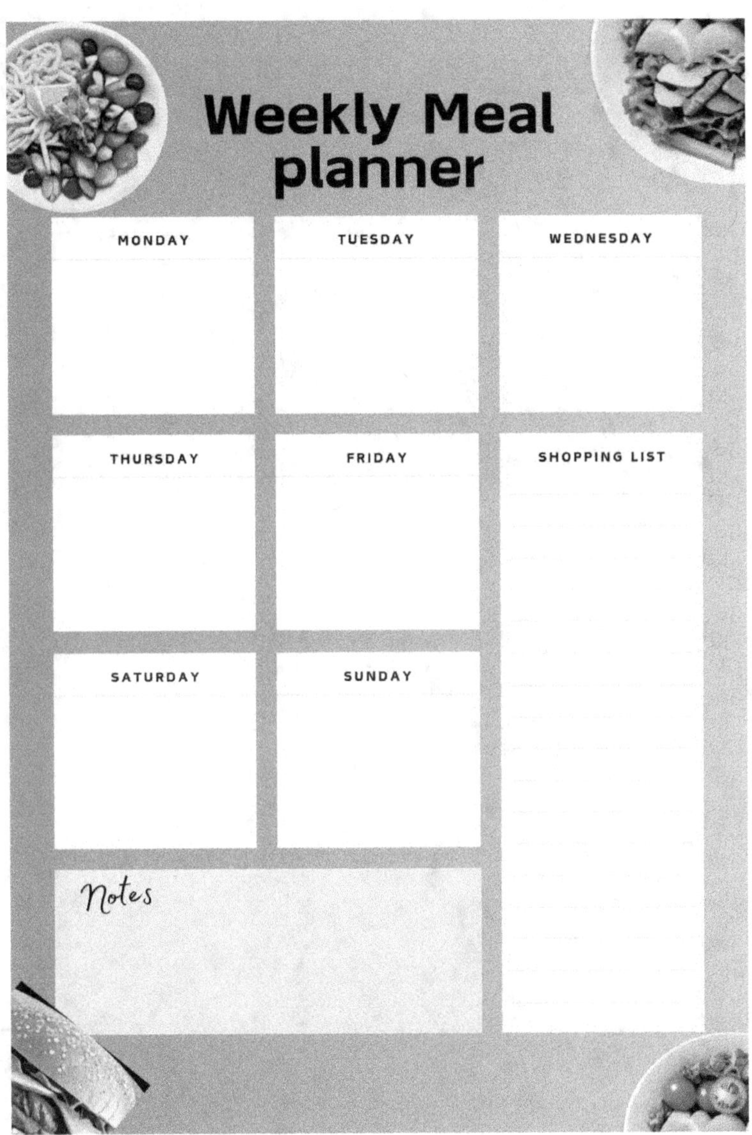

Weekly Meal planner
MONDAY
TUESDAY
WEDNESDAY
THURSDAY
FRIDAY
SHOPPING LIST
SATURDAY
SUNDAY
Notes

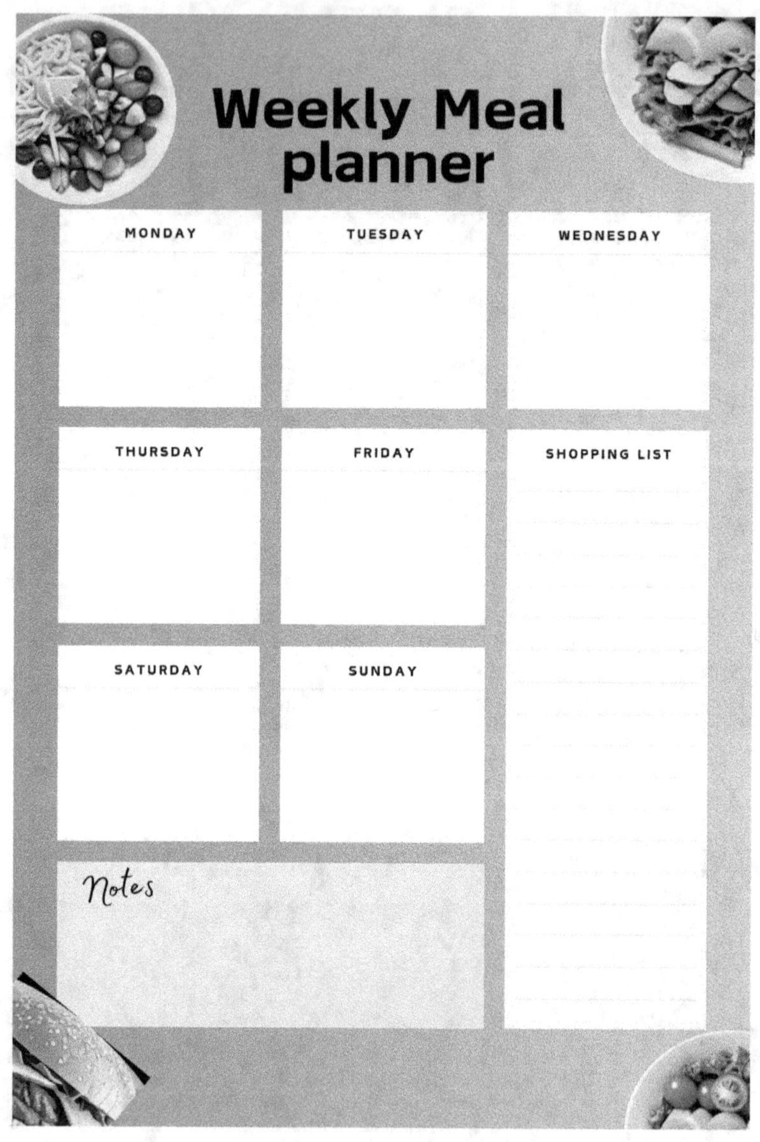

Weekly Meal planner
MONDAY
TUESDAY
WEDNESDAY
THURSDAY
FRIDAY
SHOPPING LIST
SATURDAY
SUNDAY
Notes

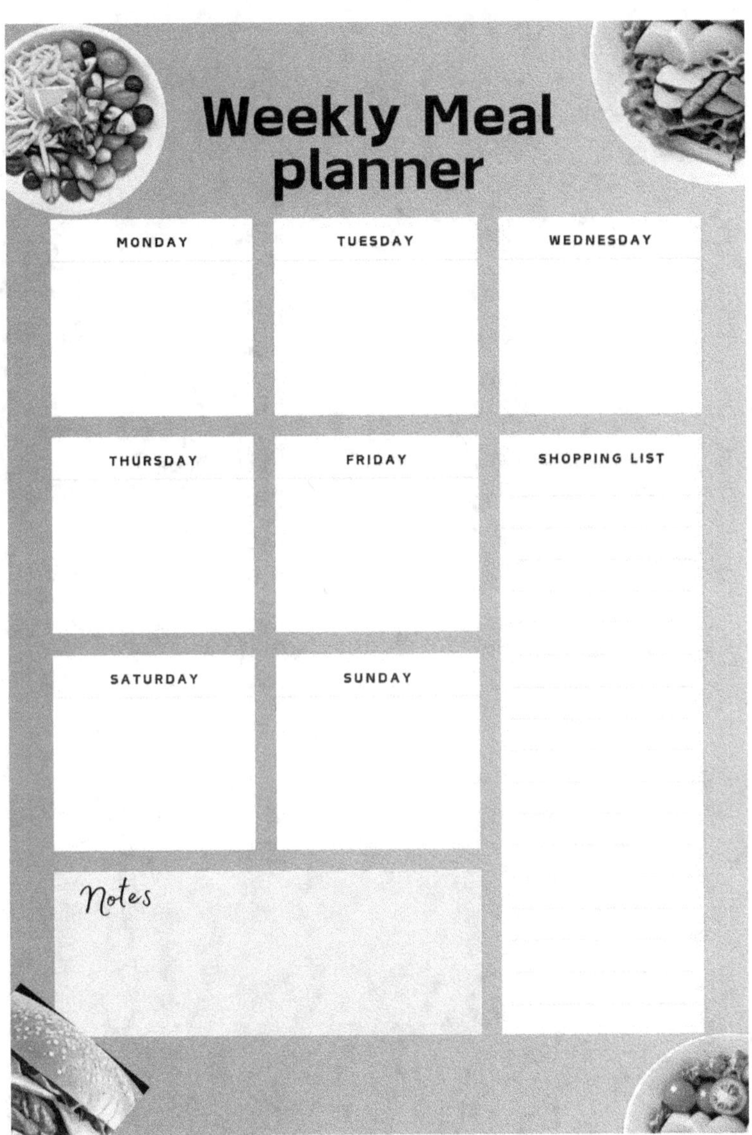

Weekly Meal planner
MONDAY
TUESDAY
WEDNESDAY
THURSDAY
FRIDAY
SHOPPING LIST
SATURDAY
SUNDAY
Notes

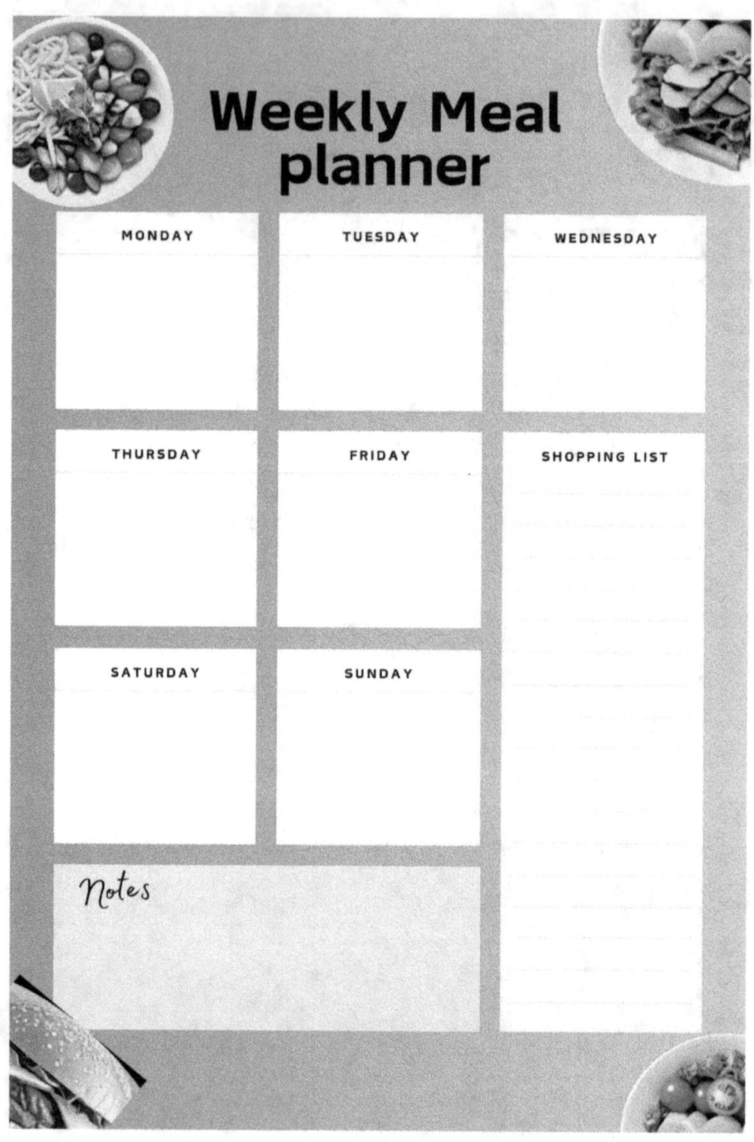

Weekly Meal planner
MONDAY
TUESDAY
WEDNESDAY
THURSDAY
FRIDAY
SHOPPING LIST
SATURDAY
SUNDAY
Notes

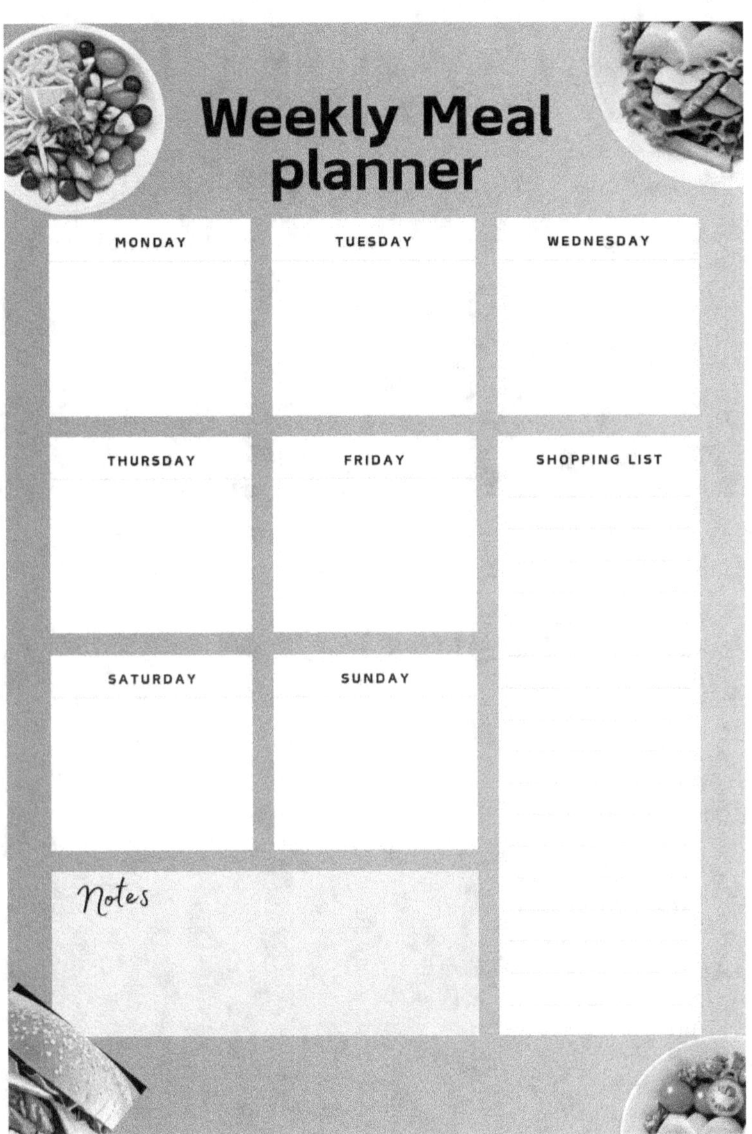

Weekly Meal planner
MONDAY
TUESDAY
WEDNESDAY
THURSDAY
FRIDAY
SHOPPING LIST
SATURDAY
SUNDAY
Notes

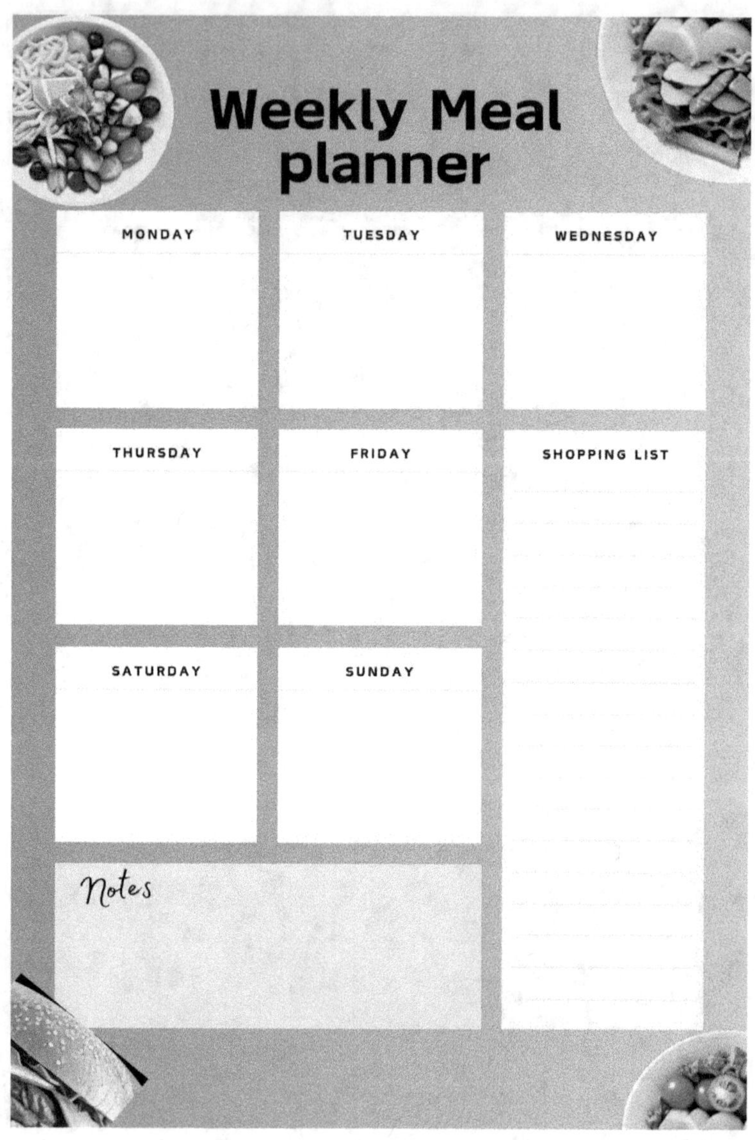

Weekly Meal planner
MONDAY
TUESDAY
WEDNESDAY
THURSDAY
FRIDAY
SHOPPING LIST
SATURDAY
SUNDAY
Notes

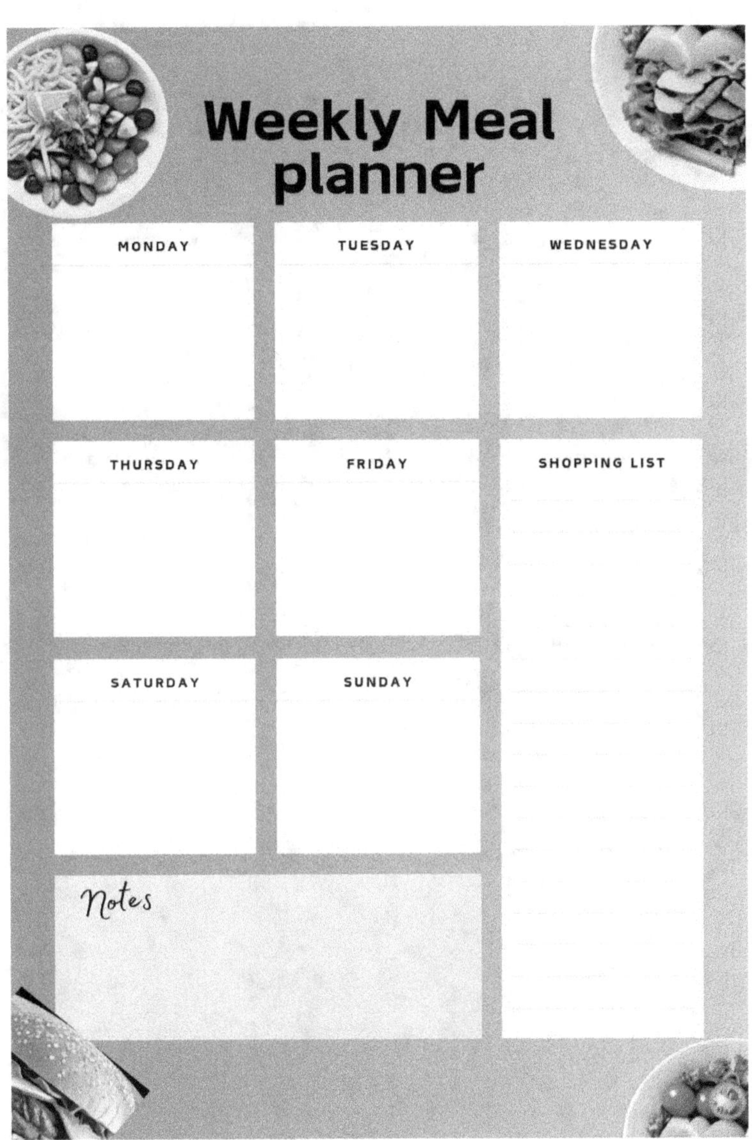

Weekly Meal planner

MONDAY

TUESDAY

WEDNESDAY

THURSDAY

FRIDAY

SHOPPING LIST

SATURDAY

SUNDAY

Notes

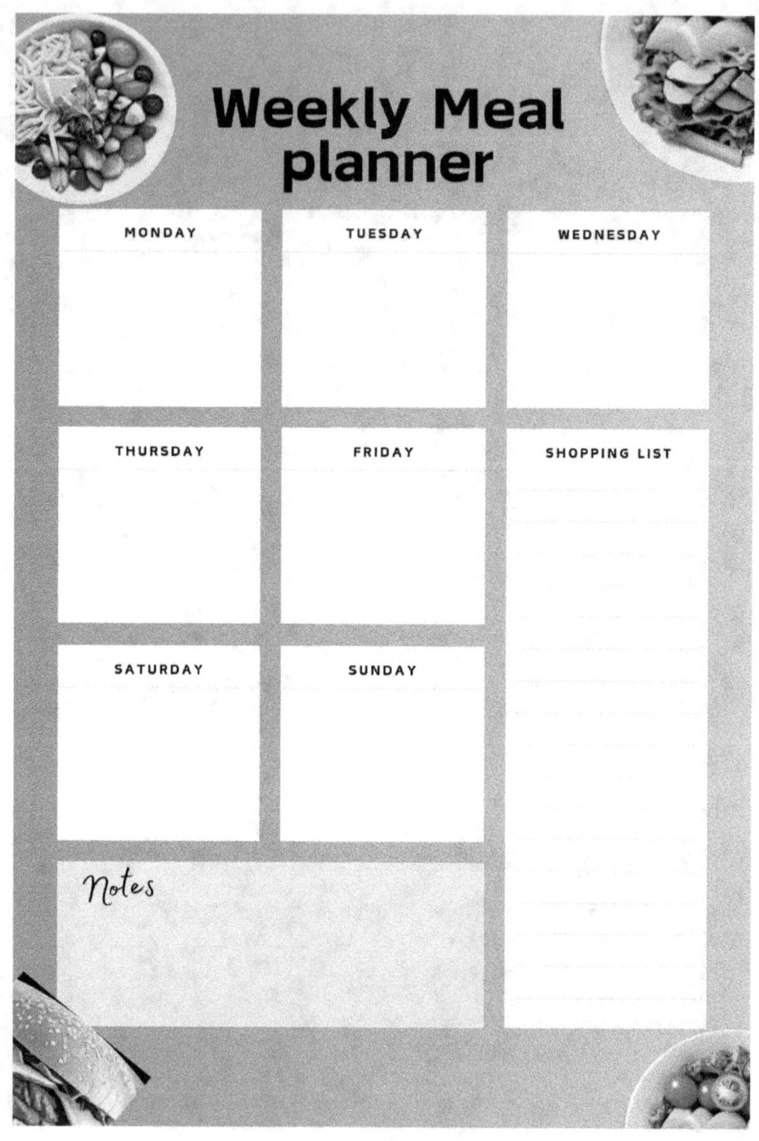

Weekly Meal planner
MONDAY
TUESDAY
WEDNESDAY
THURSDAY
FRIDAY
SHOPPING LIST
SATURDAY
SUNDAY
Notes

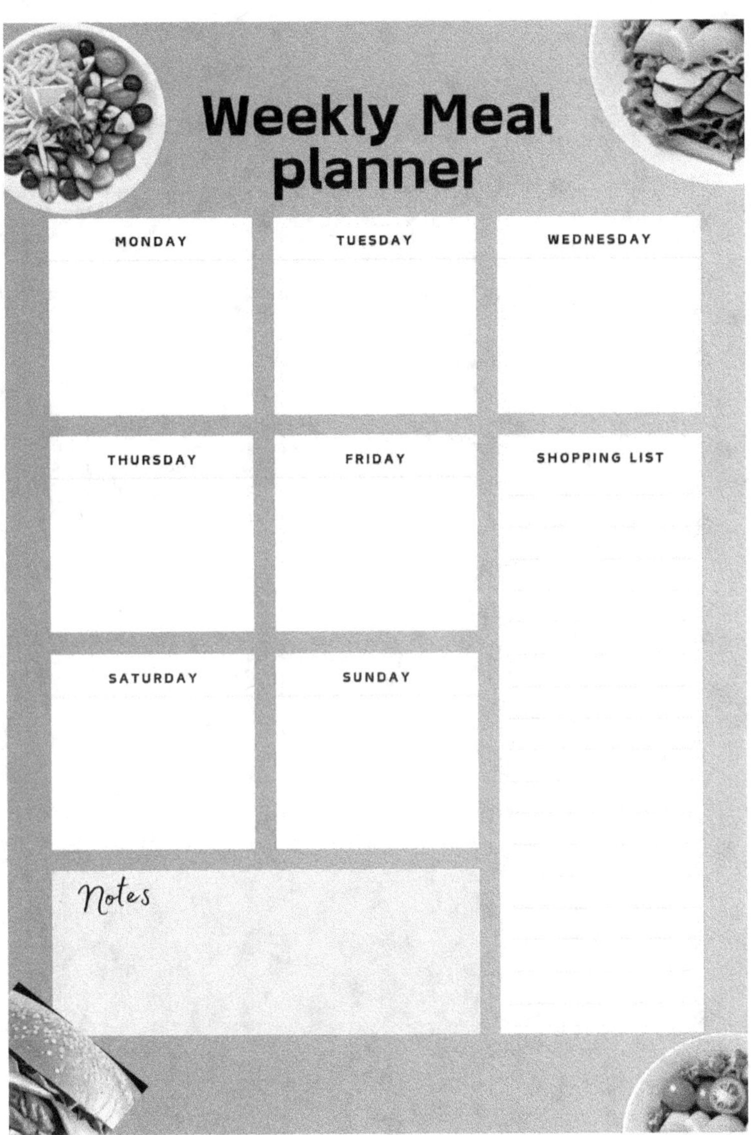

194

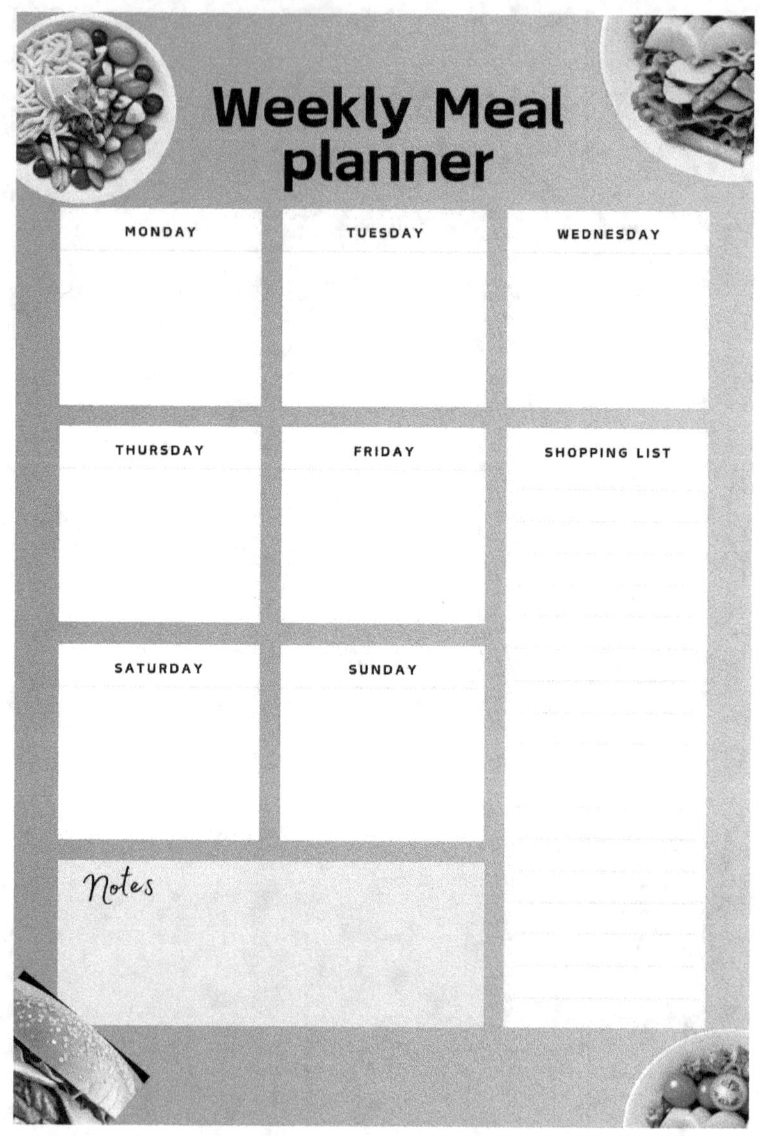

Weekly Meal planner
MONDAY
TUESDAY
WEDNESDAY
THURSDAY
FRIDAY
SHOPPING LIST
SATURDAY
SUNDAY
Notes

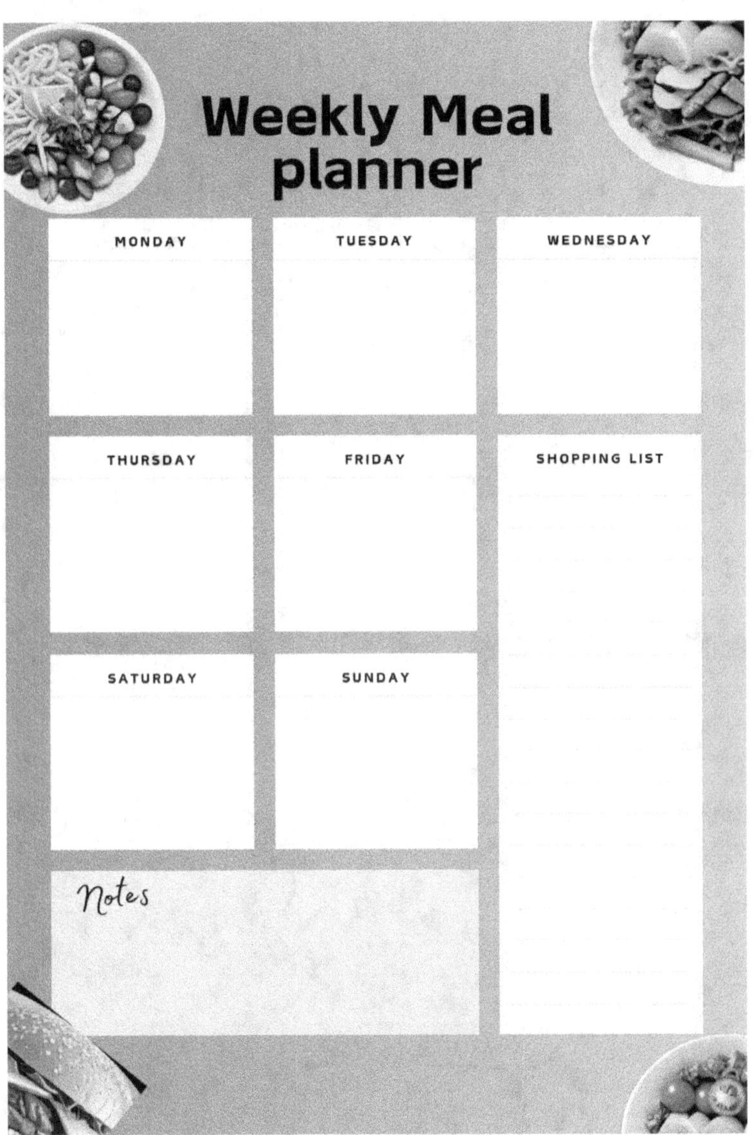

Weekly Meal planner
MONDAY
TUESDAY
WEDNESDAY
THURSDAY
FRIDAY
SHOPPING LIST
SATURDAY
SUNDAY
Notes

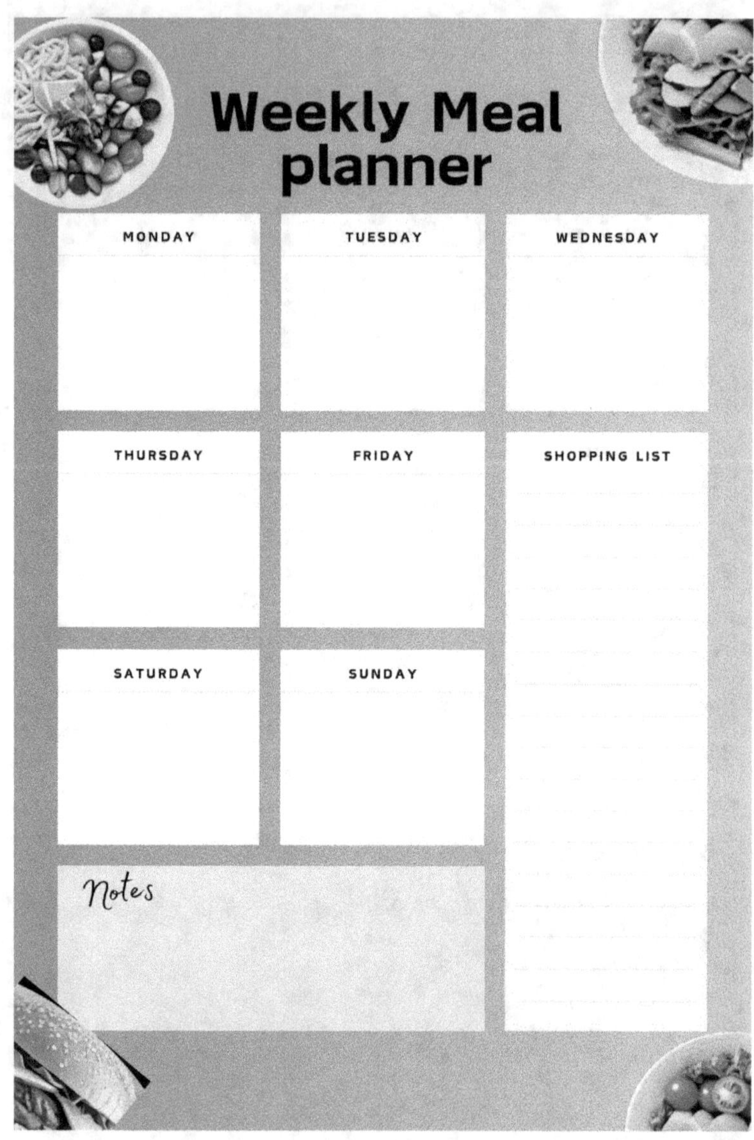

197

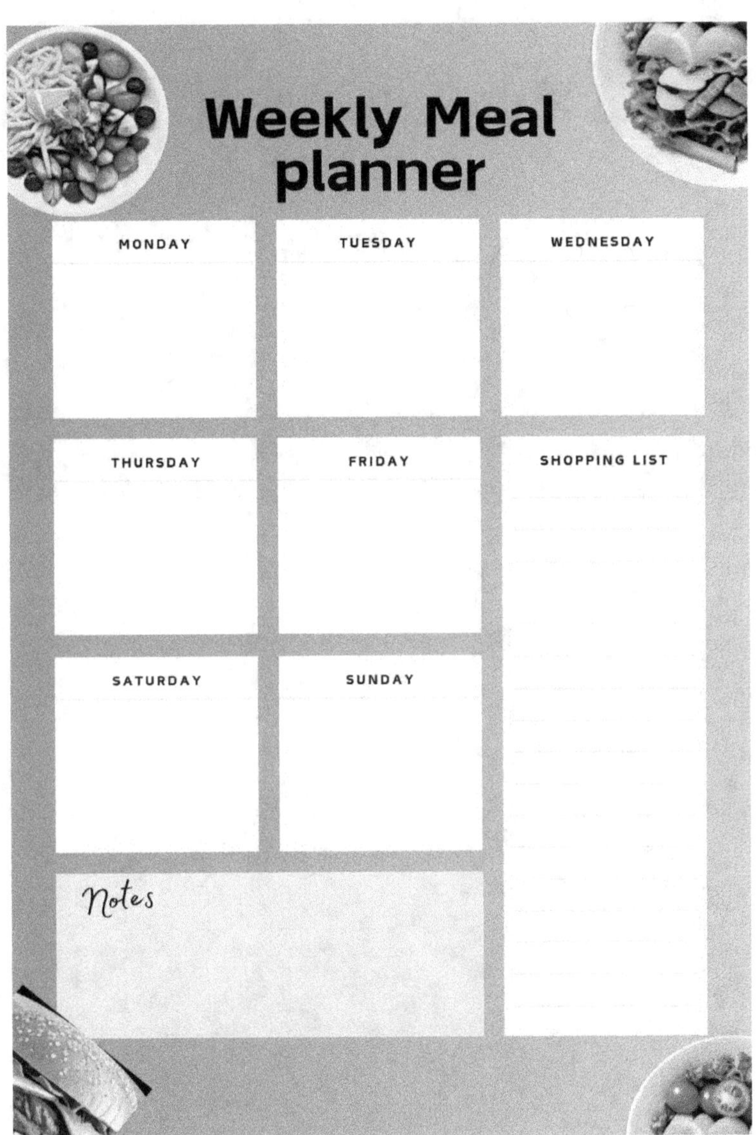

Weekly Meal planner
MONDAY
TUESDAY
WEDNESDAY
THURSDAY
FRIDAY
SHOPPING LIST
SATURDAY
SUNDAY
Notes

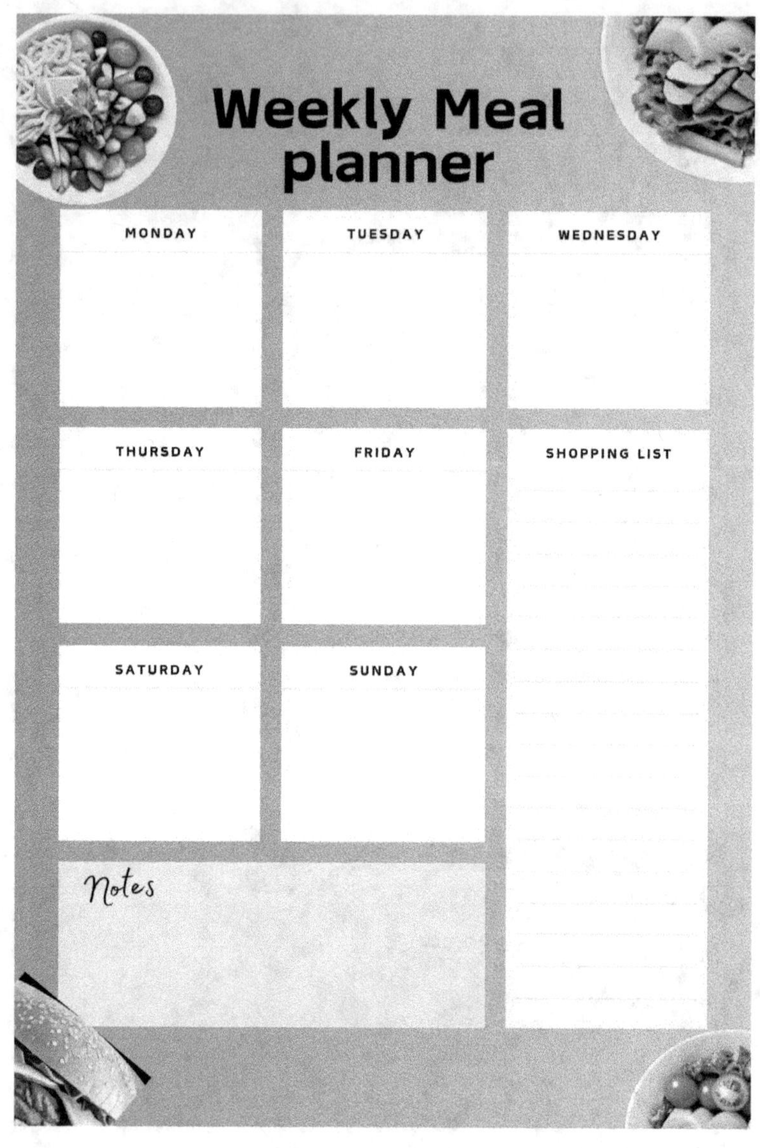

Weekly Meal planner
MONDAY
TUESDAY
WEDNESDAY
THURSDAY
FRIDAY
SHOPPING LIST
SATURDAY
SUNDAY
Notes

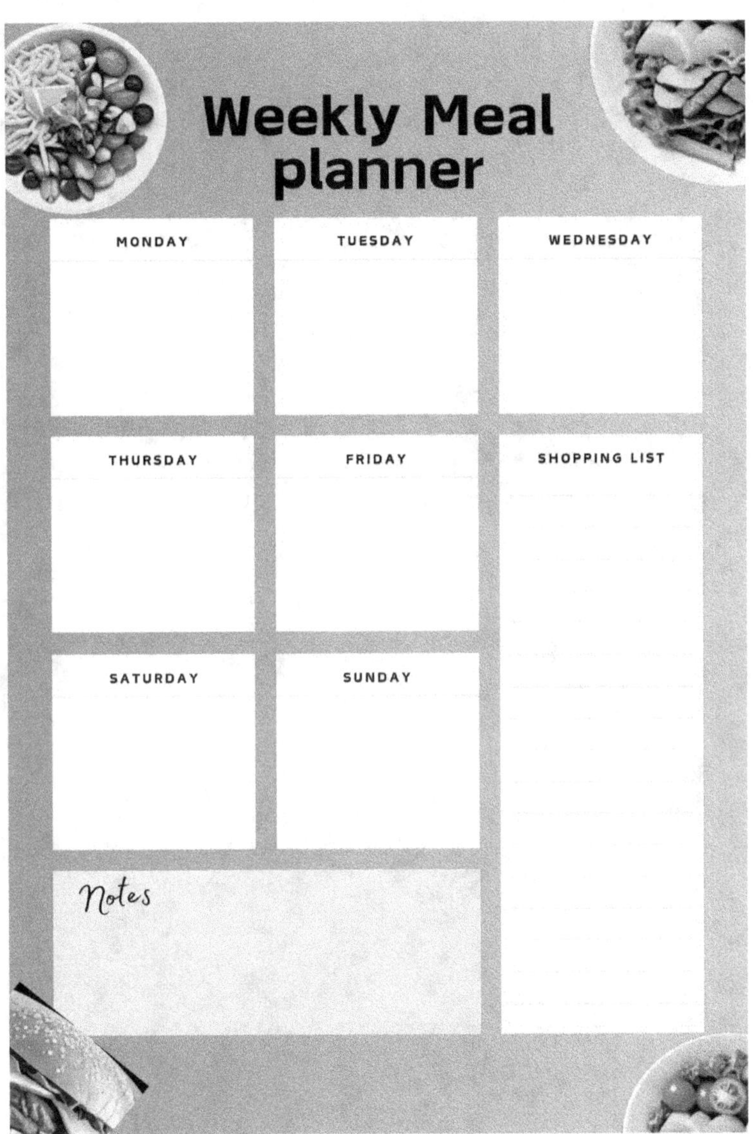

Weekly Meal planner
MONDAY
TUESDAY
WEDNESDAY
THURSDAY
FRIDAY
SHOPPING LIST
SATURDAY
SUNDAY
Notes

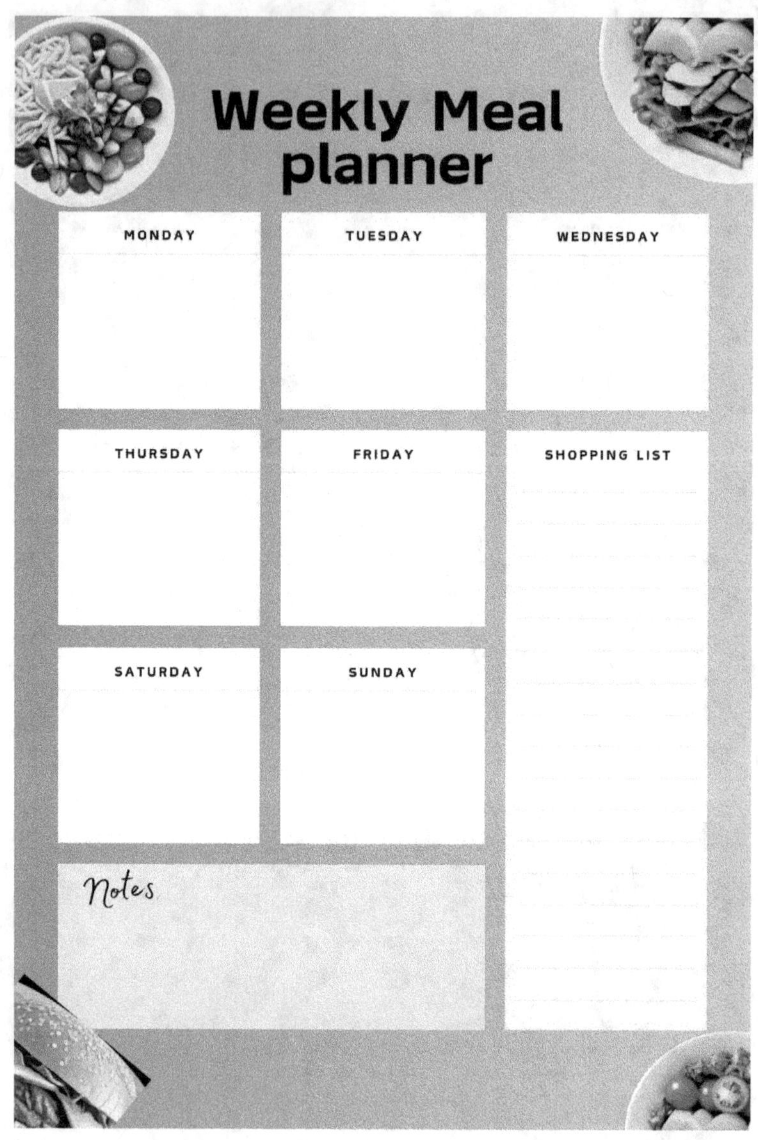

Weekly Meal planner
MONDAY
TUESDAY
WEDNESDAY
THURSDAY
FRIDAY
SHOPPING LIST
SATURDAY
SUNDAY
Notes

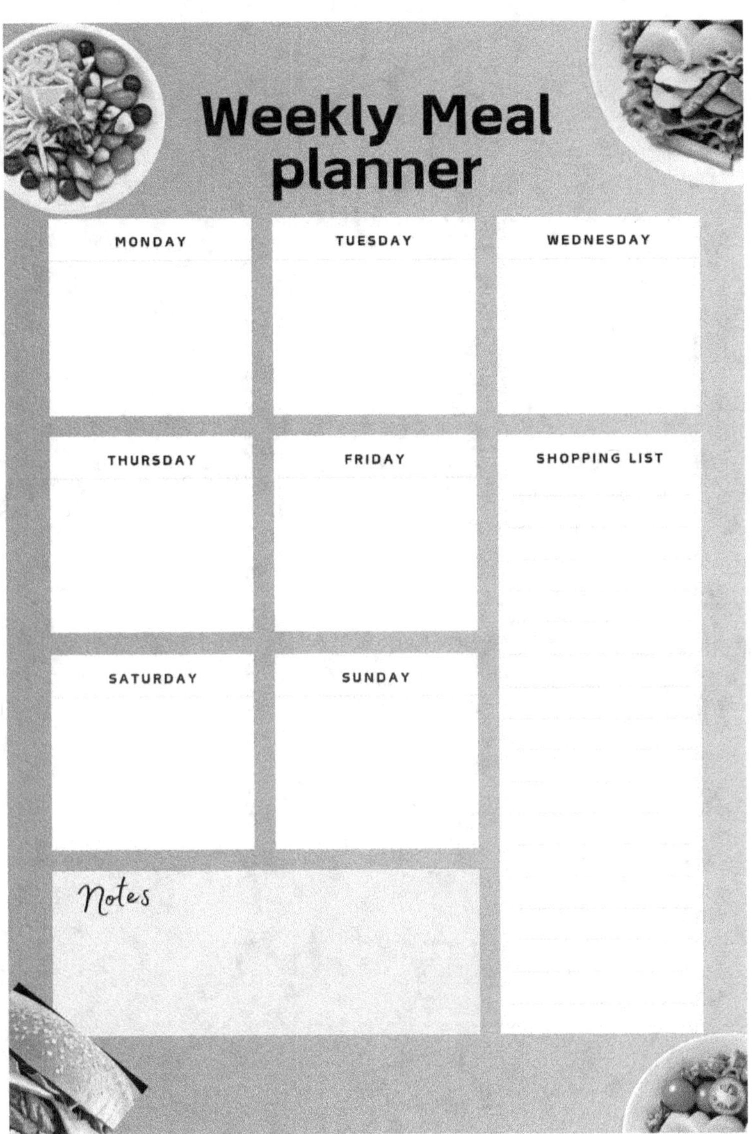

Weekly Meal planner
MONDAY
TUESDAY
WEDNESDAY
THURSDAY
FRIDAY
SHOPPING LIST
SATURDAY
SUNDAY
Notes

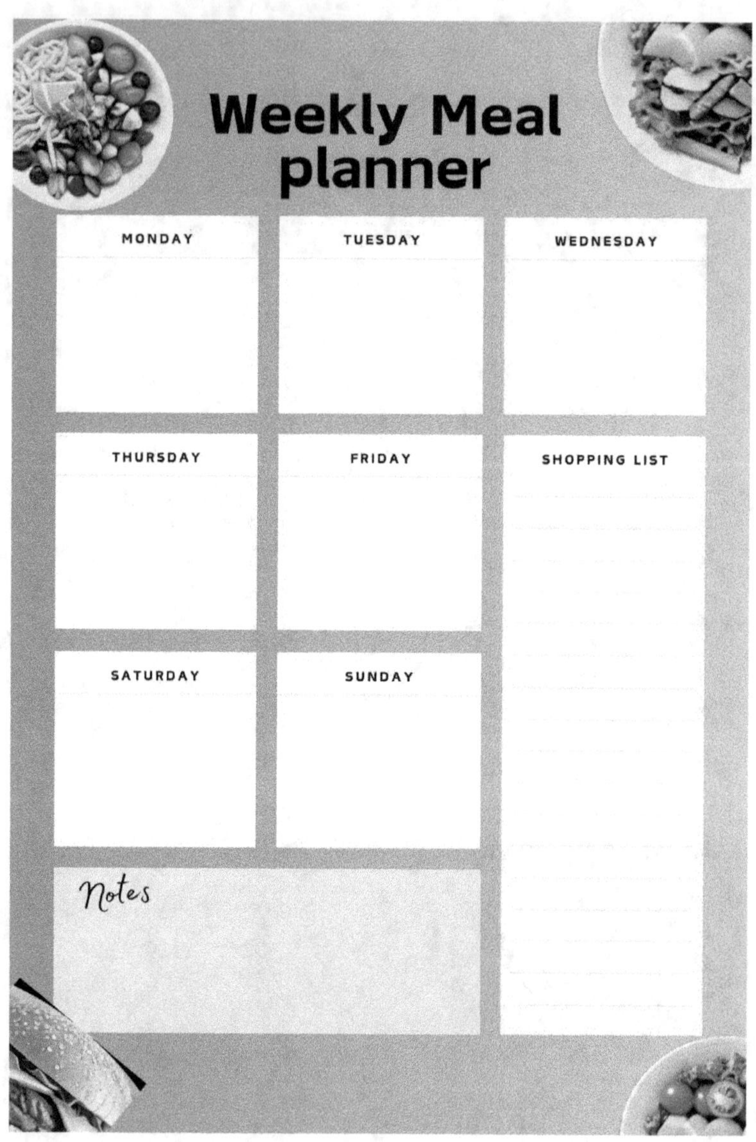

Weekly Meal planner
MONDAY
TUESDAY
WEDNESDAY
THURSDAY
FRIDAY
SHOPPING LIST
SATURDAY
SUNDAY
Notes

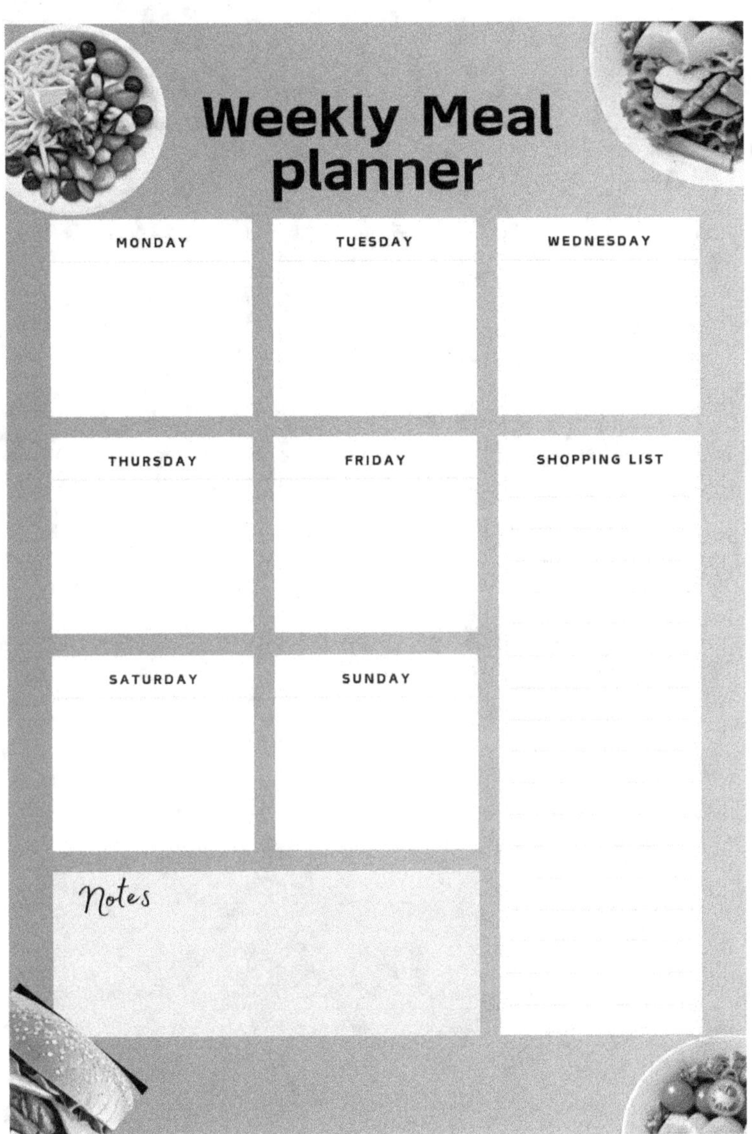

Weekly Meal planner
MONDAY
TUESDAY
WEDNESDAY
THURSDAY
FRIDAY
SHOPPING LIST
SATURDAY
SUNDAY
Notes

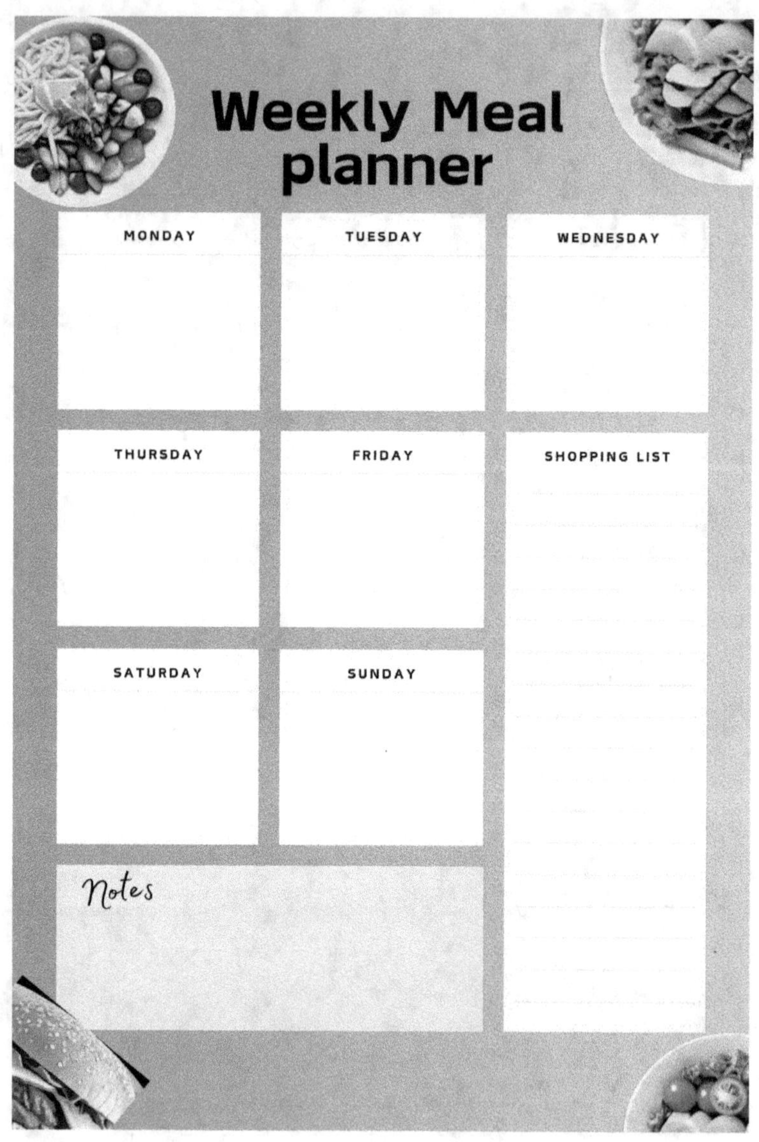

Weekly Meal planner
MONDAY
TUESDAY
WEDNESDAY
THURSDAY
FRIDAY
SHOPPING LIST
SATURDAY
SUNDAY
Notes

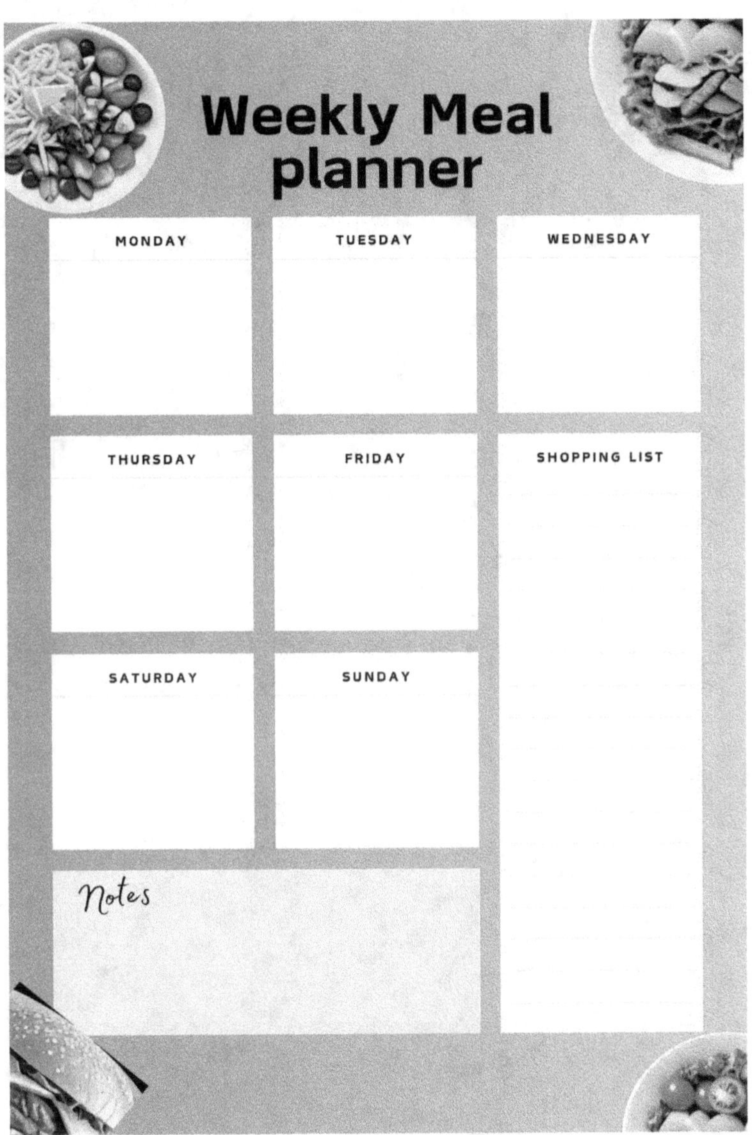

Weekly Meal planner
MONDAY
TUESDAY
WEDNESDAY
THURSDAY
FRIDAY
SHOPPING LIST
SATURDAY
SUNDAY
Notes

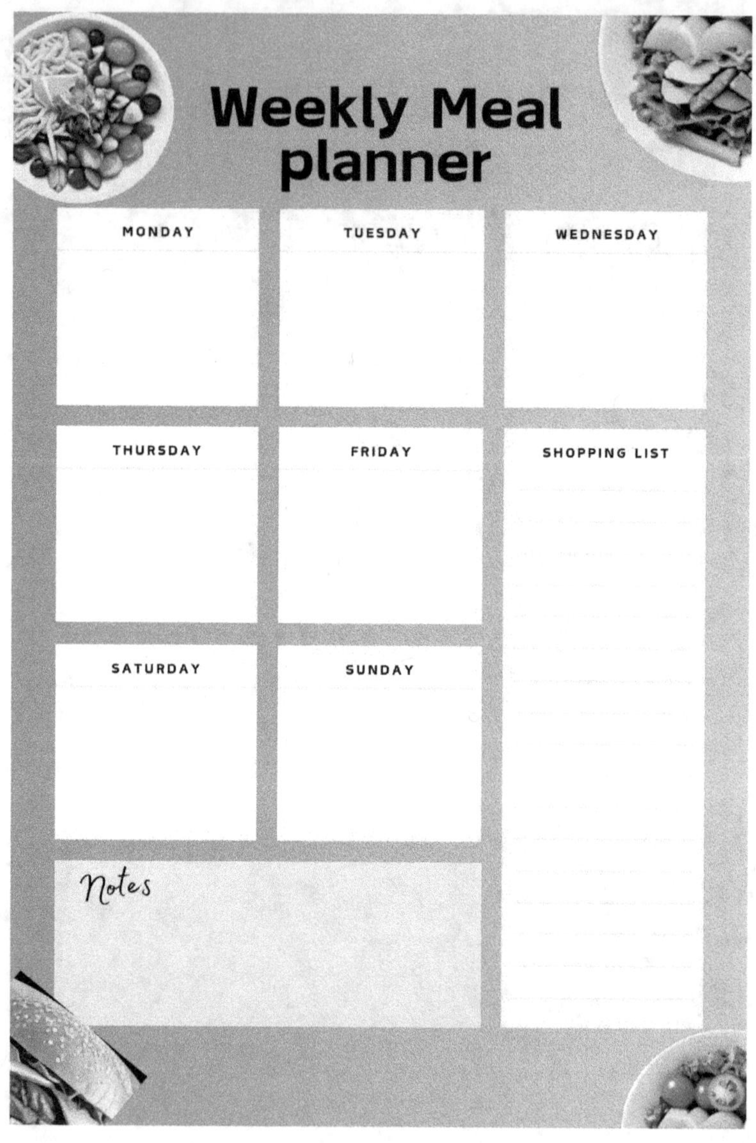

Weekly Meal planner
MONDAY
TUESDAY
WEDNESDAY
THURSDAY
FRIDAY
SHOPPING LIST
SATURDAY
SUNDAY
Notes

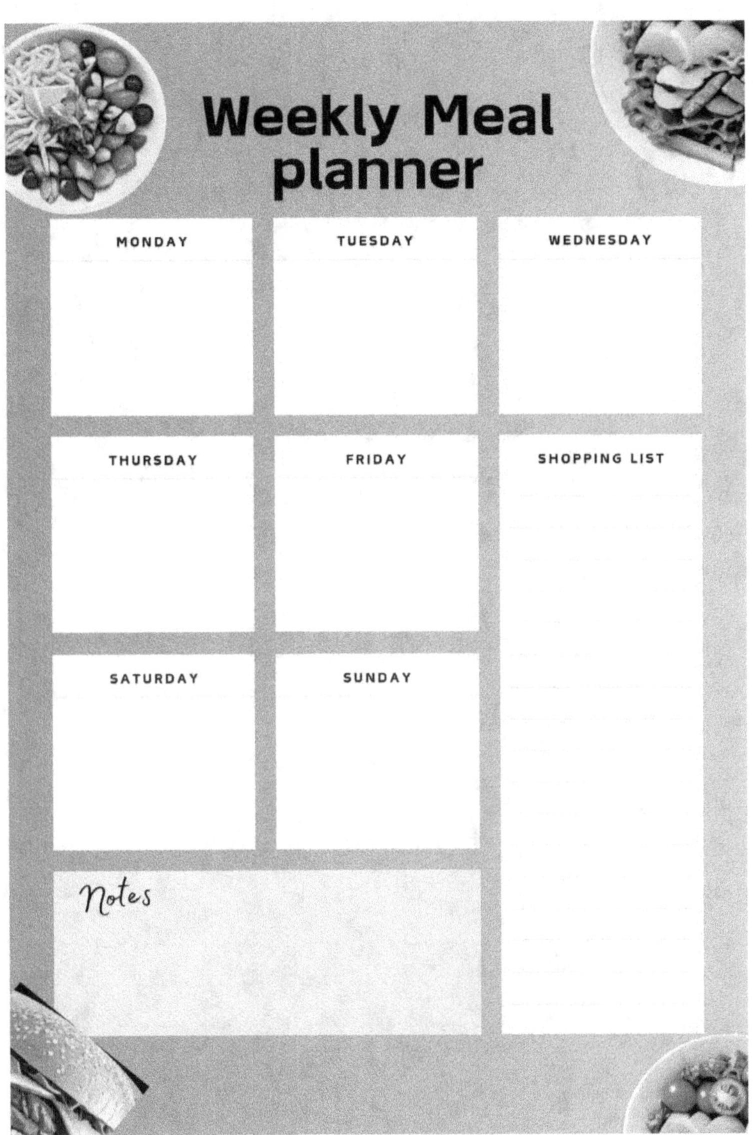
Weekly Meal planner
MONDAY
TUESDAY
WEDNESDAY
THURSDAY
FRIDAY
SHOPPING LIST
SATURDAY
SUNDAY
Notes

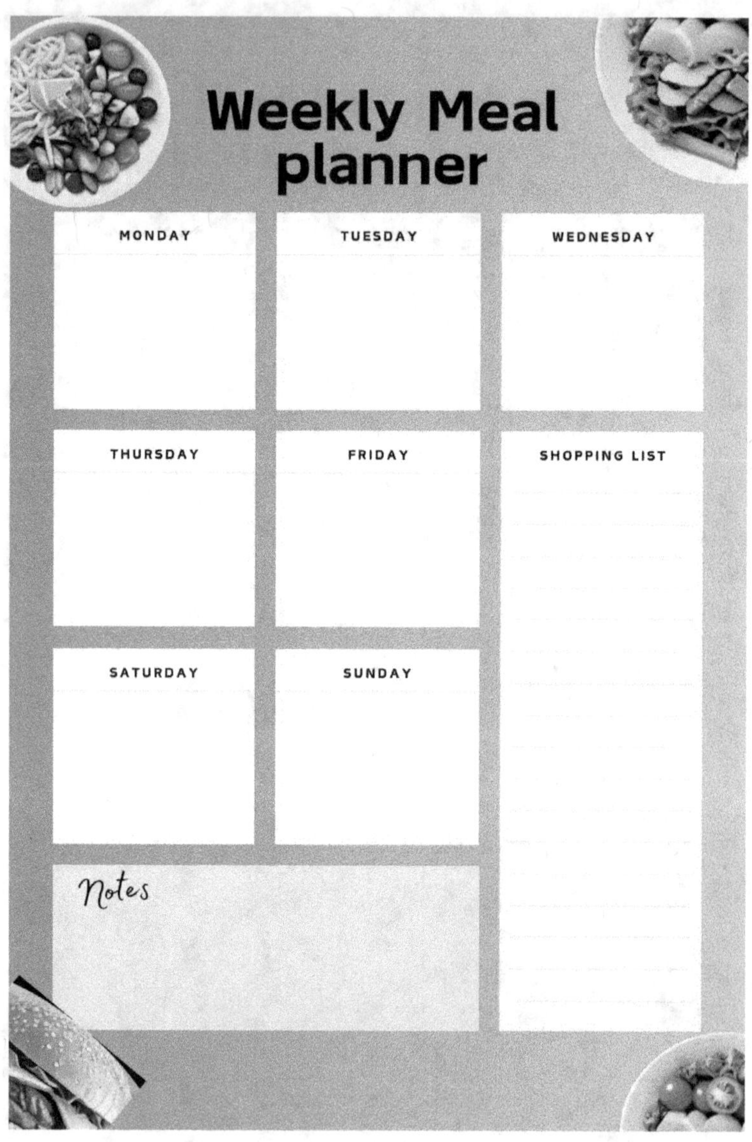

Weekly Meal
planner
MONDAY
TUESDAY
WEDNESDAY
THURSDAY
FRIDAY
SHOPPING LIST
SATURDAY
SUNDAY
Notes

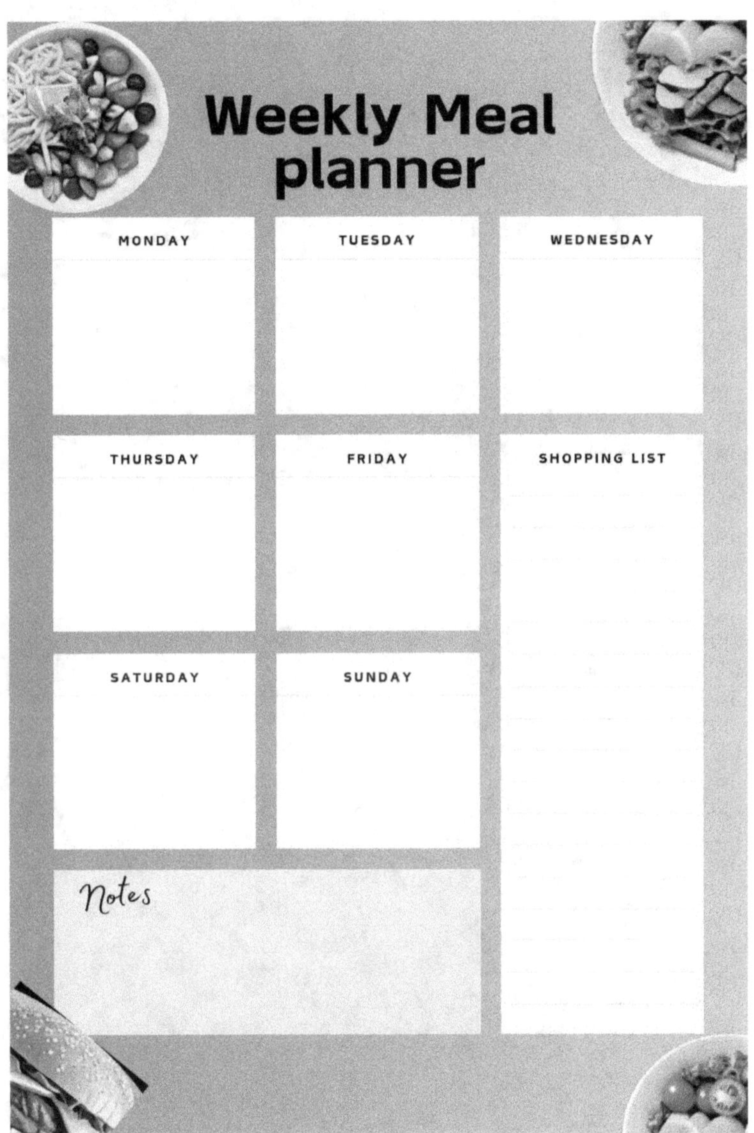

Weekly Meal planner
MONDAY
TUESDAY
WEDNESDAY
THURSDAY
FRIDAY
SHOPPING LIST
SATURDAY
SUNDAY
Notes

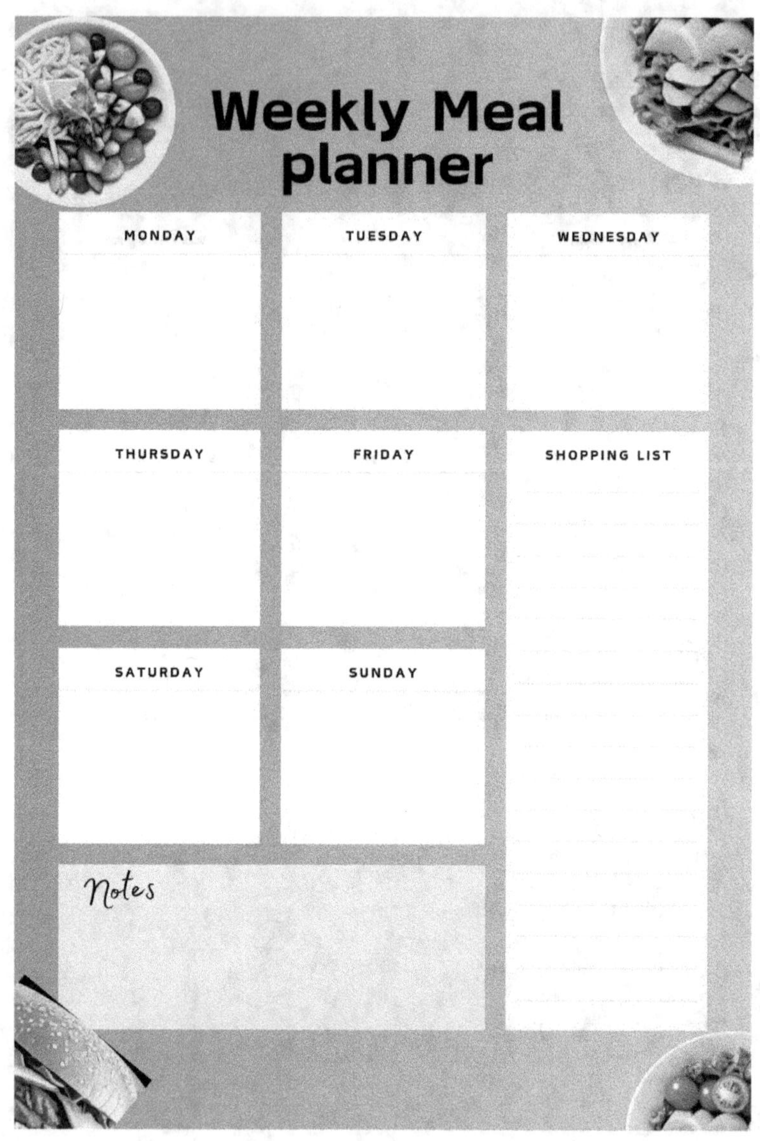

Weekly Meal planner
MONDAY
TUESDAY
WEDNESDAY
THURSDAY
FRIDAY
SHOPPING LIST
SATURDAY
SUNDAY
Notes

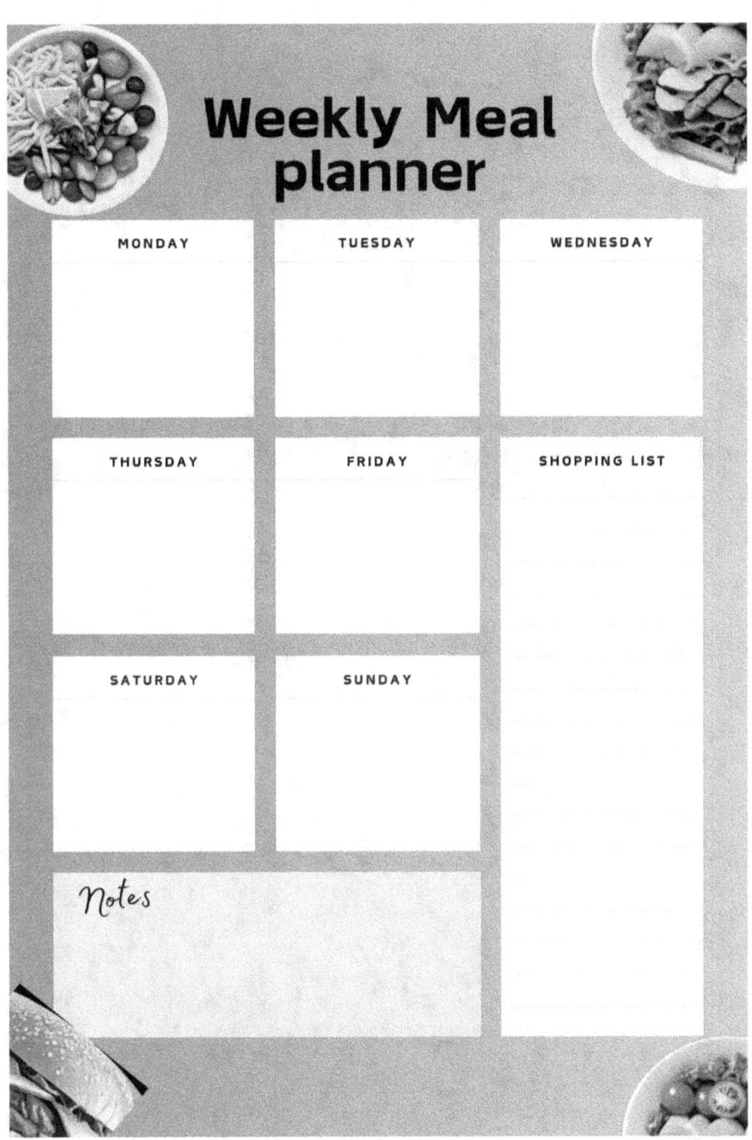

Weekly Meal planner

MONDAY
TUESDAY
WEDNESDAY
THURSDAY
FRIDAY
SHOPPING LIST
SATURDAY
SUNDAY
Notes

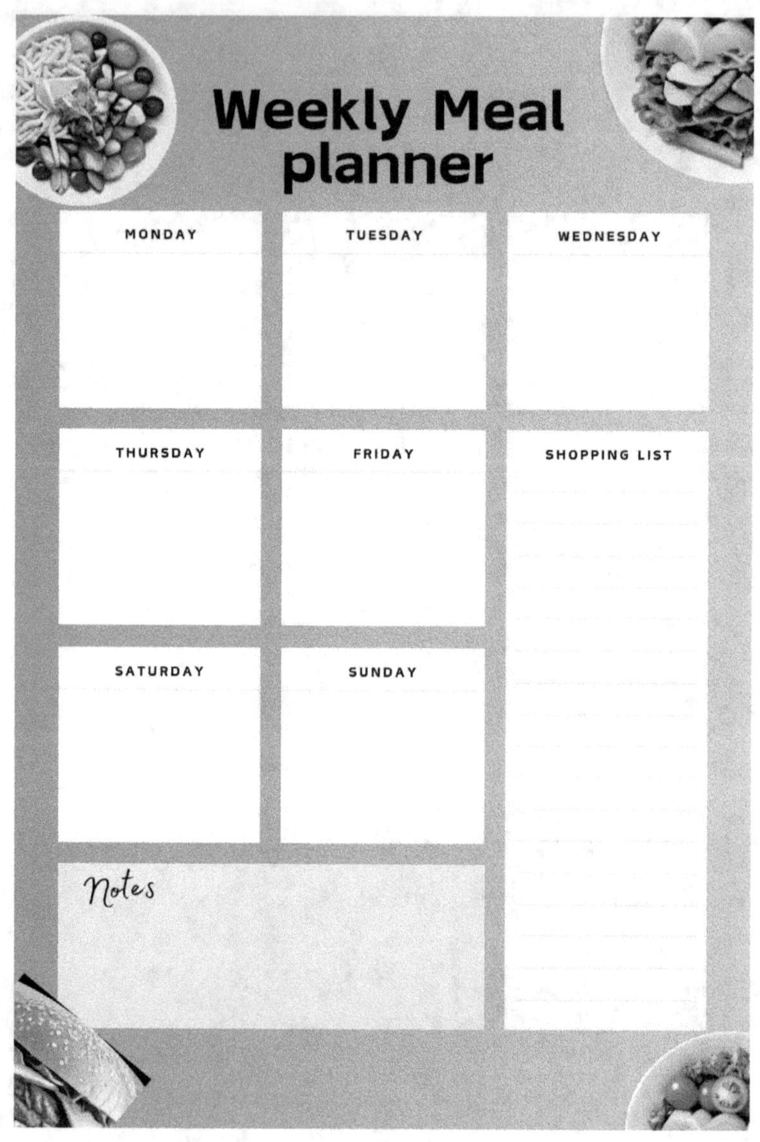

213

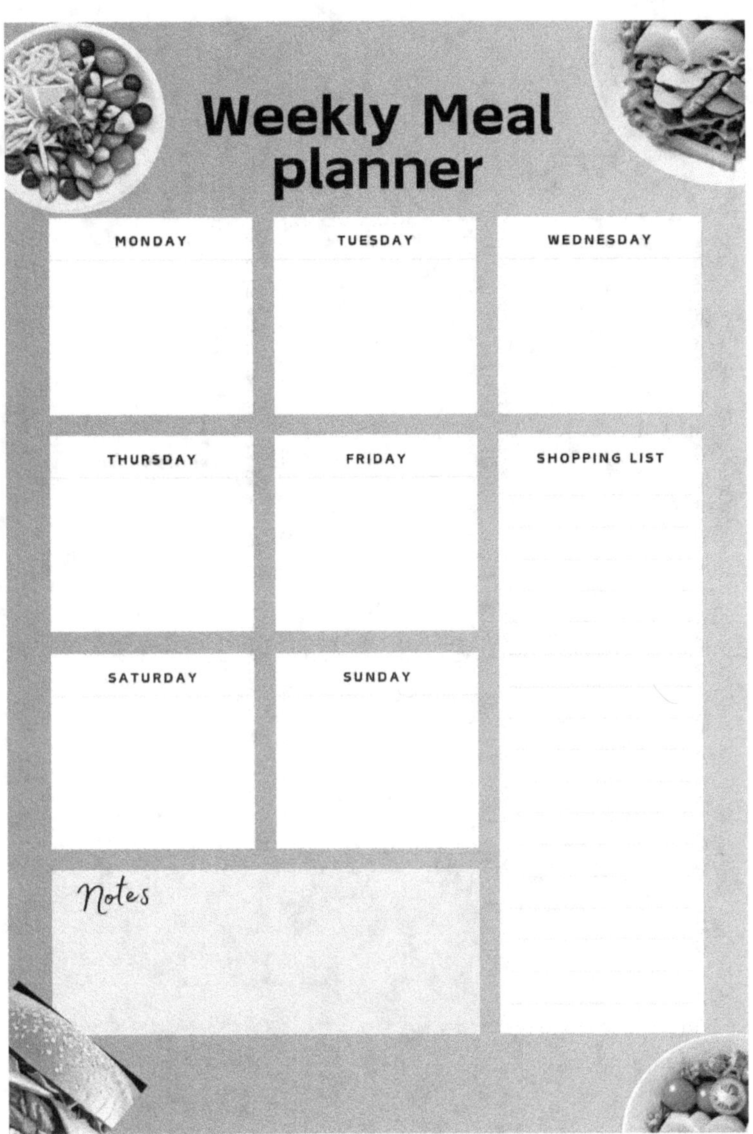

Weekly Meal planner
MONDAY
TUESDAY
WEDNESDAY
THURSDAY
FRIDAY
SHOPPING LIST
SATURDAY
SUNDAY
Notes

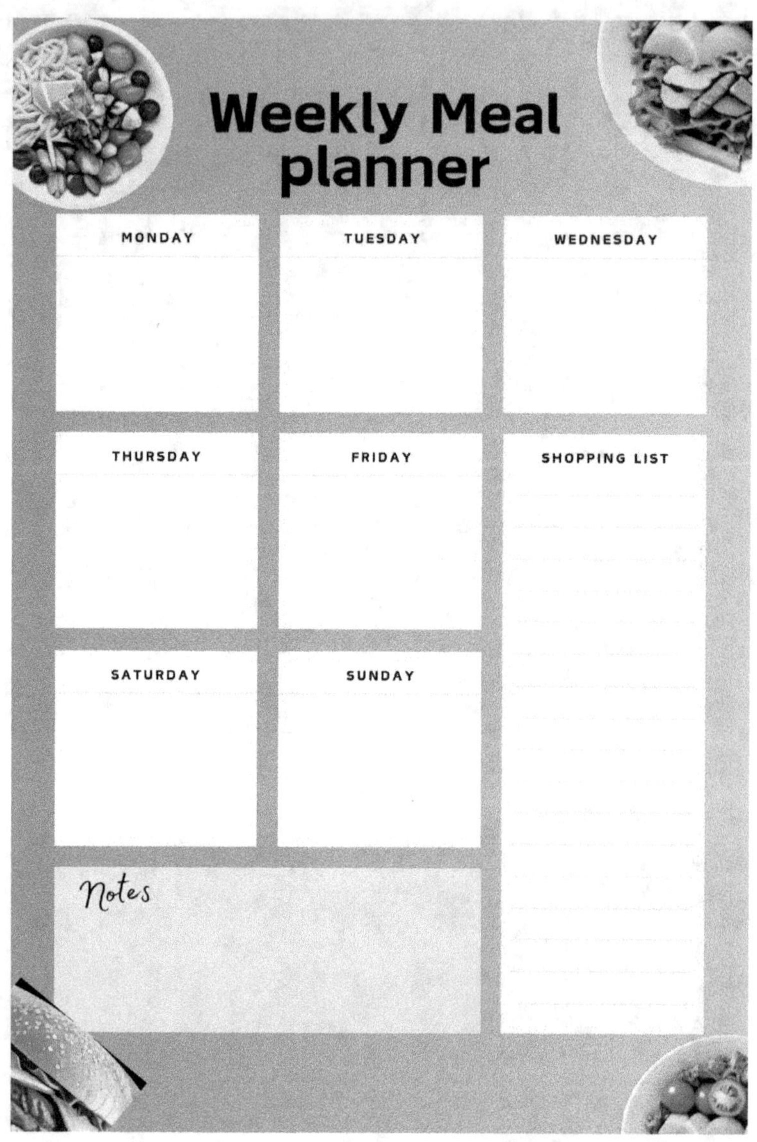

Weekly Meal planner
MONDAY
TUESDAY
WEDNESDAY
THURSDAY
FRIDAY
SHOPPING LIST
SATURDAY
SUNDAY
Notes

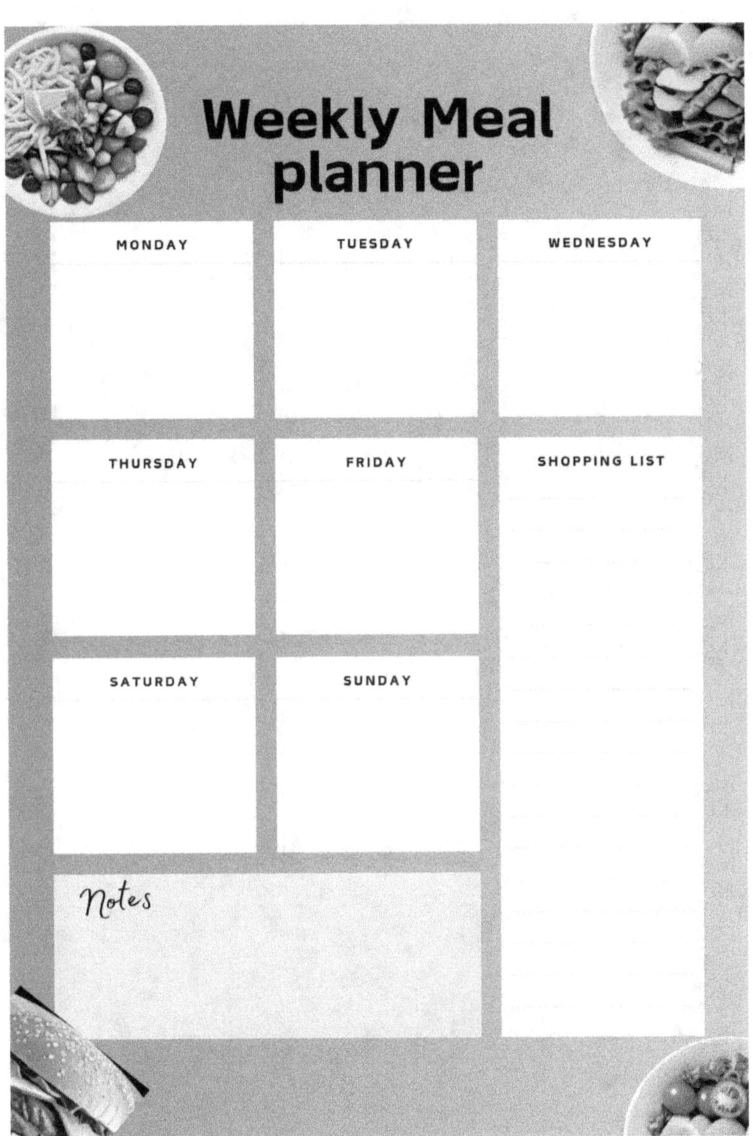
Weekly Meal planner
MONDAY
TUESDAY
WEDNESDAY
THURSDAY
FRIDAY
SHOPPING LIST
SATURDAY
SUNDAY
Notes

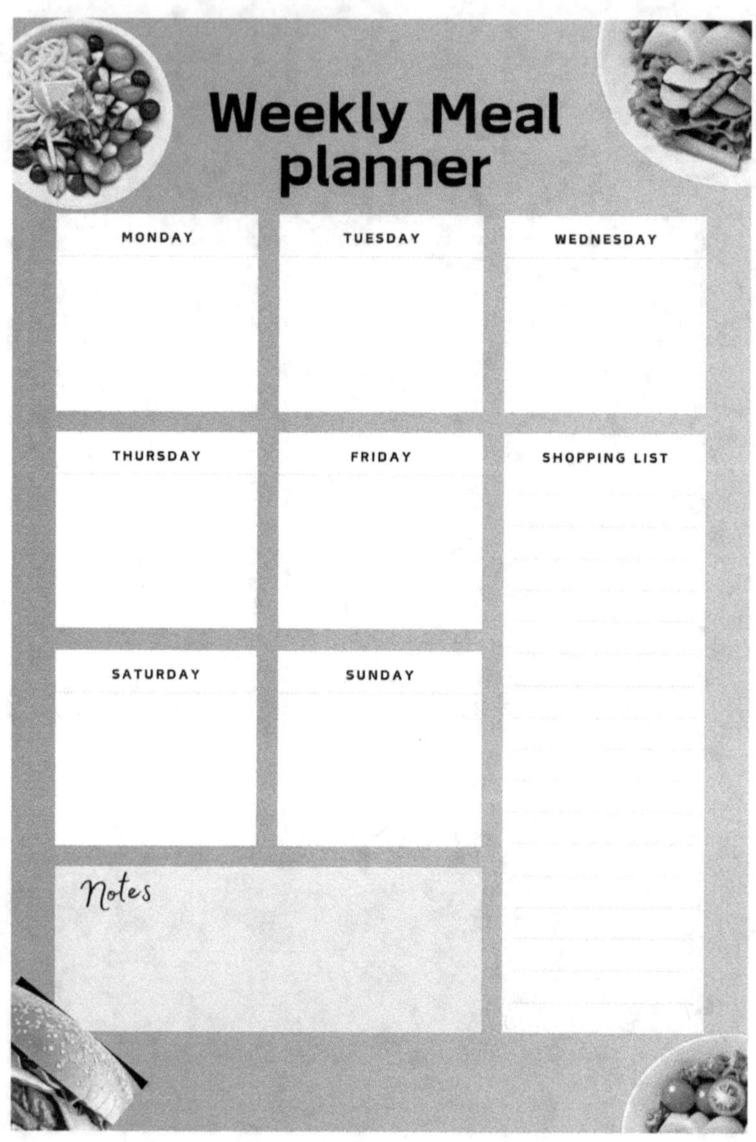

Weekly Meal planner
MONDAY
TUESDAY
WEDNESDAY
THURSDAY
FRIDAY
SHOPPING LIST
SATURDAY
SUNDAY
Notes

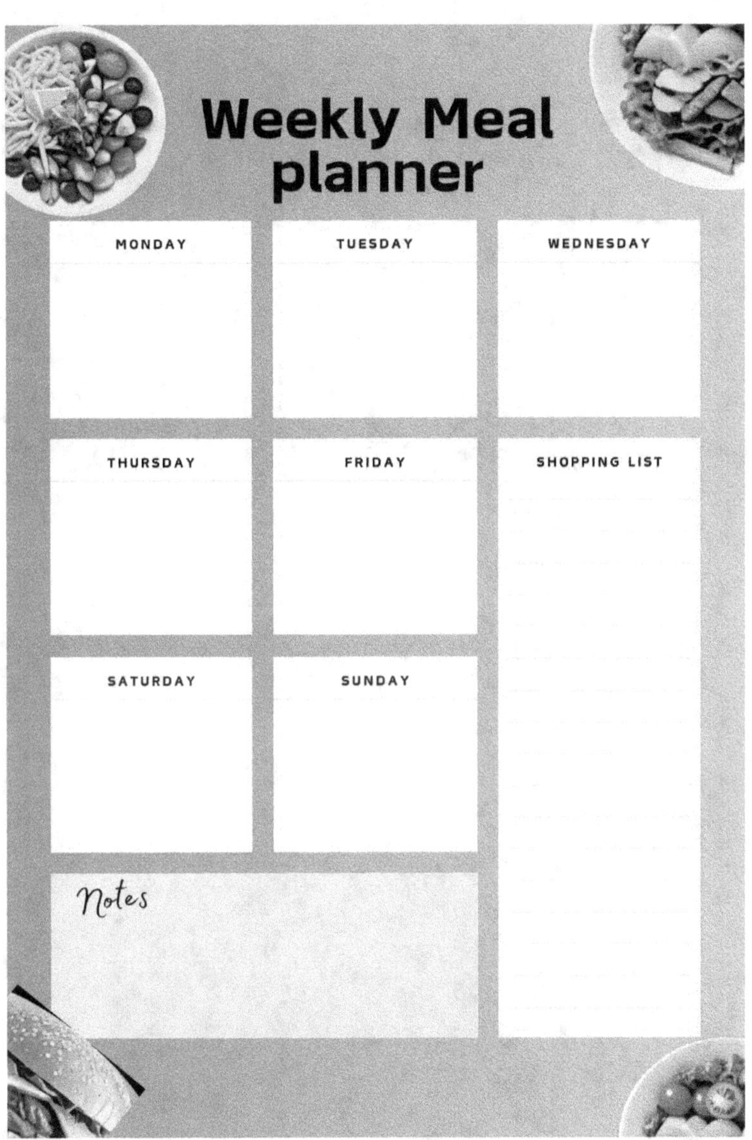

Weekly Meal planner
MONDAY
TUESDAY
WEDNESDAY
THURSDAY
FRIDAY
SHOPPING LIST
SATURDAY
SUNDAY
Notes

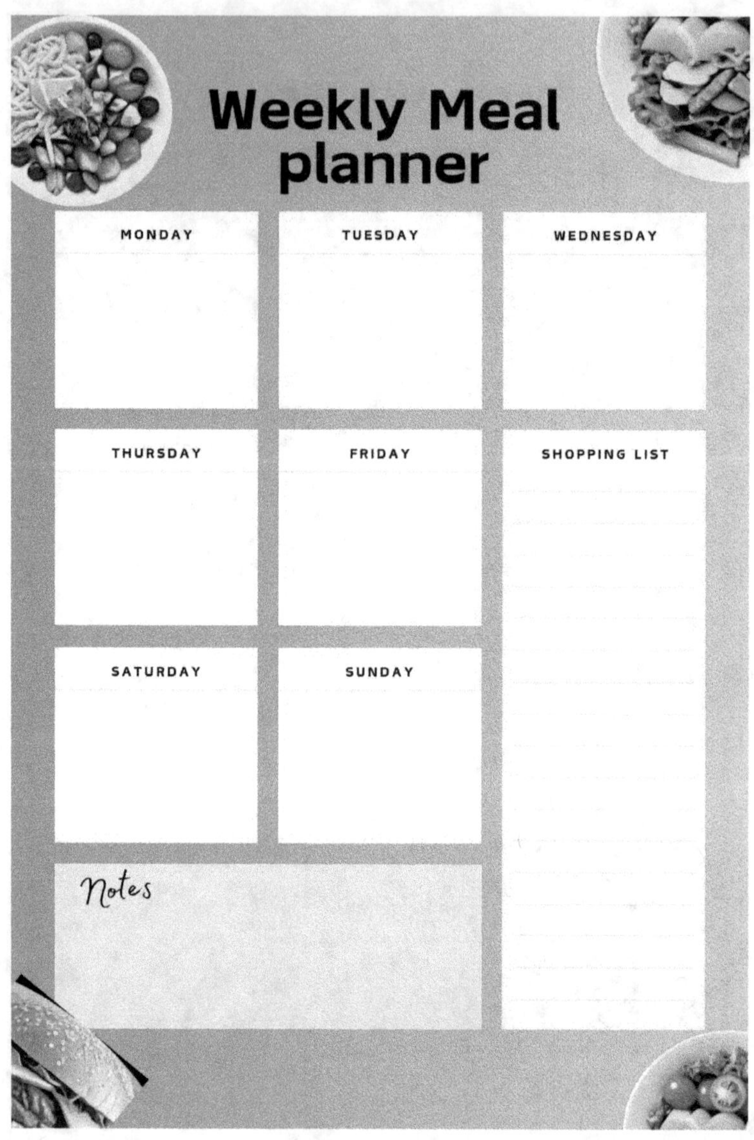

Weekly Meal planner
MONDAY
TUESDAY
WEDNESDAY
THURSDAY
FRIDAY
SHOPPING LIST
SATURDAY
SUNDAY
Notes

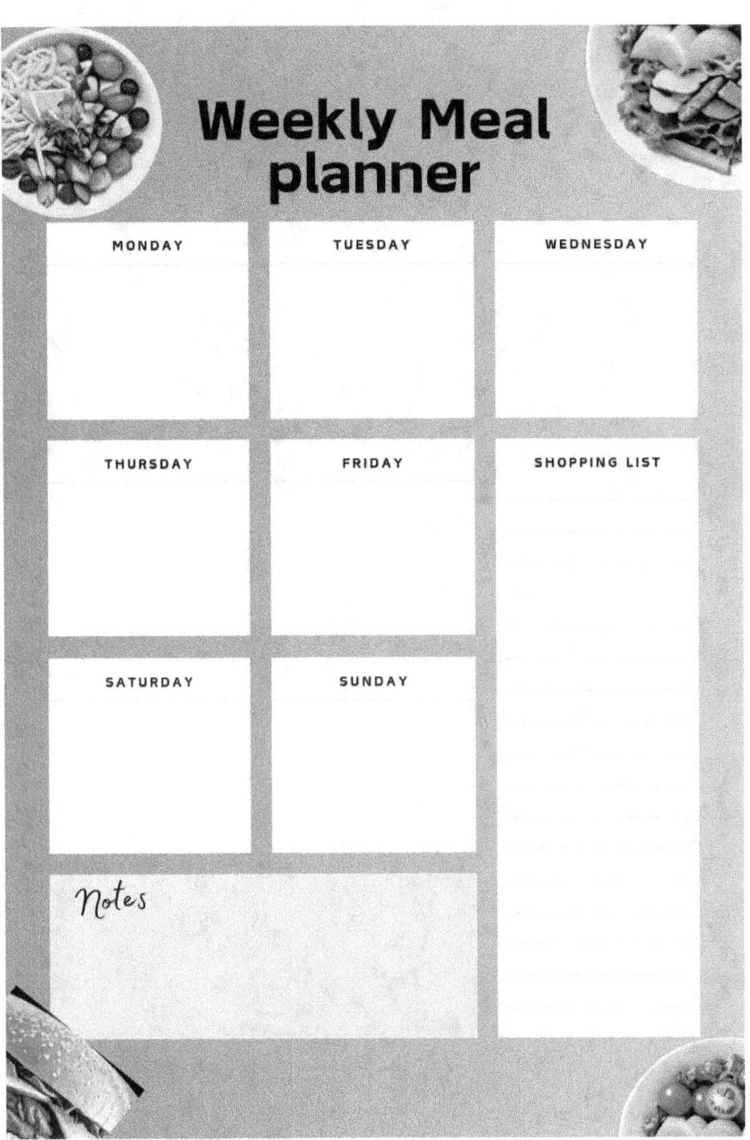
Weekly Meal planner
MONDAY
TUESDAY
WEDNESDAY
THURSDAY
FRIDAY
SHOPPING LIST
SATURDAY
SUNDAY
Notes

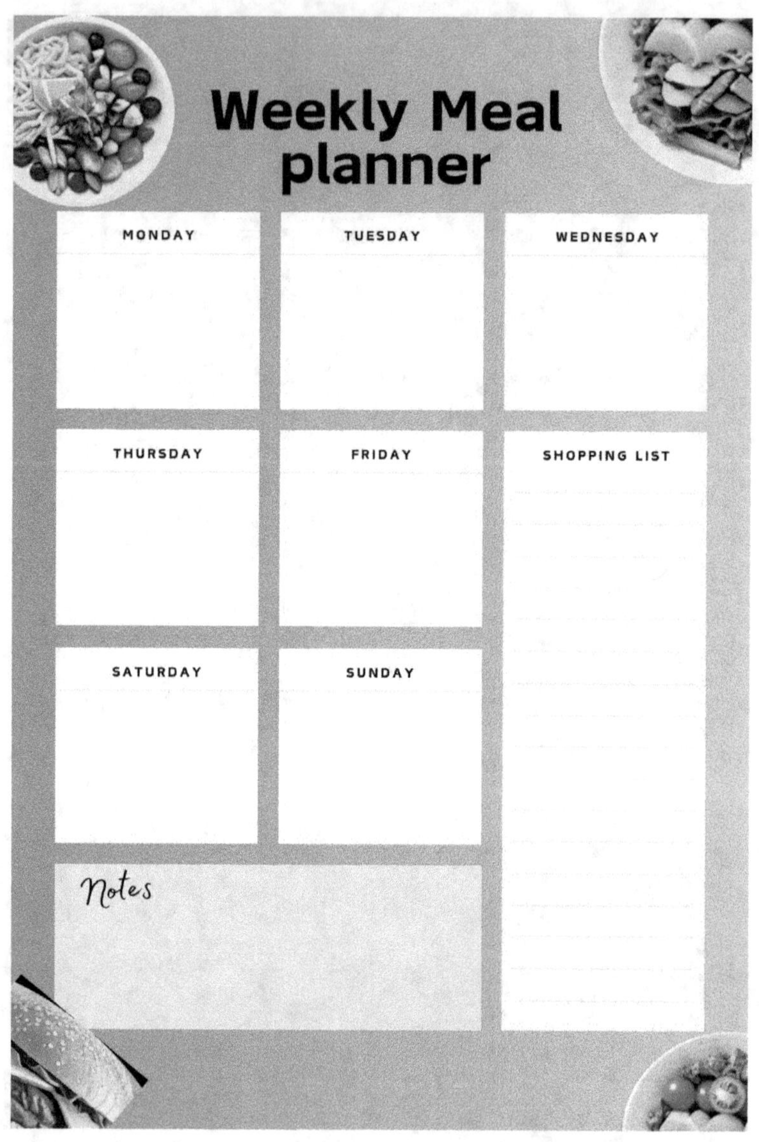

Weekly Meal planner
MONDAY
TUESDAY
WEDNESDAY
THURSDAY
FRIDAY
SHOPPING LIST
SATURDAY
SUNDAY
Notes

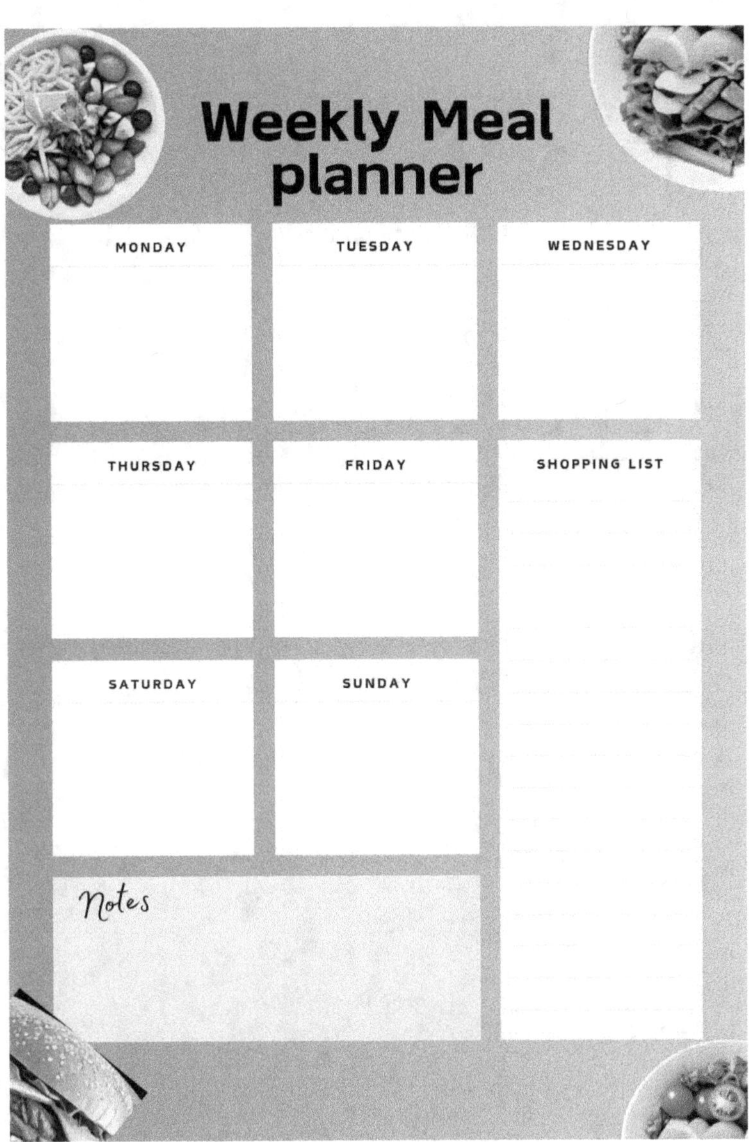

Weekly Meal planner
MONDAY
TUESDAY
WEDNESDAY
THURSDAY
FRIDAY
SHOPPING LIST
SATURDAY
SUNDAY
Notes

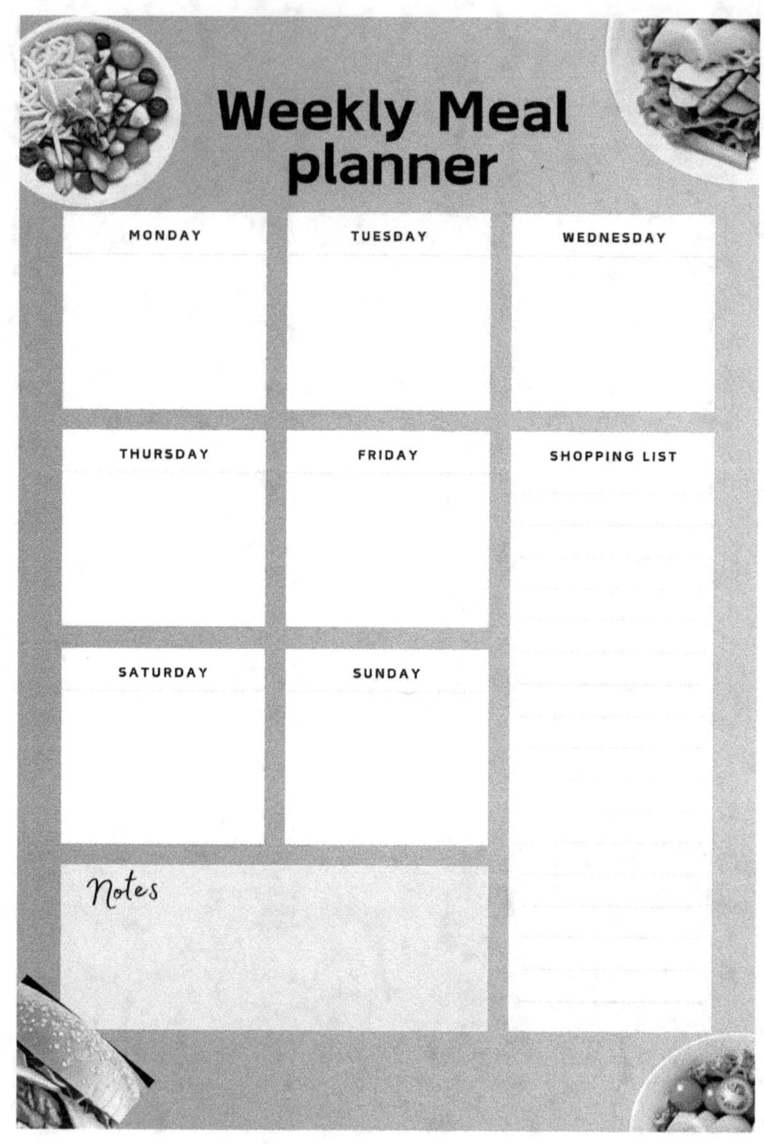

Weekly Meal planner
MONDAY
TUESDAY
WEDNESDAY
THURSDAY
FRIDAY
SHOPPING LIST
SATURDAY
SUNDAY
Notes

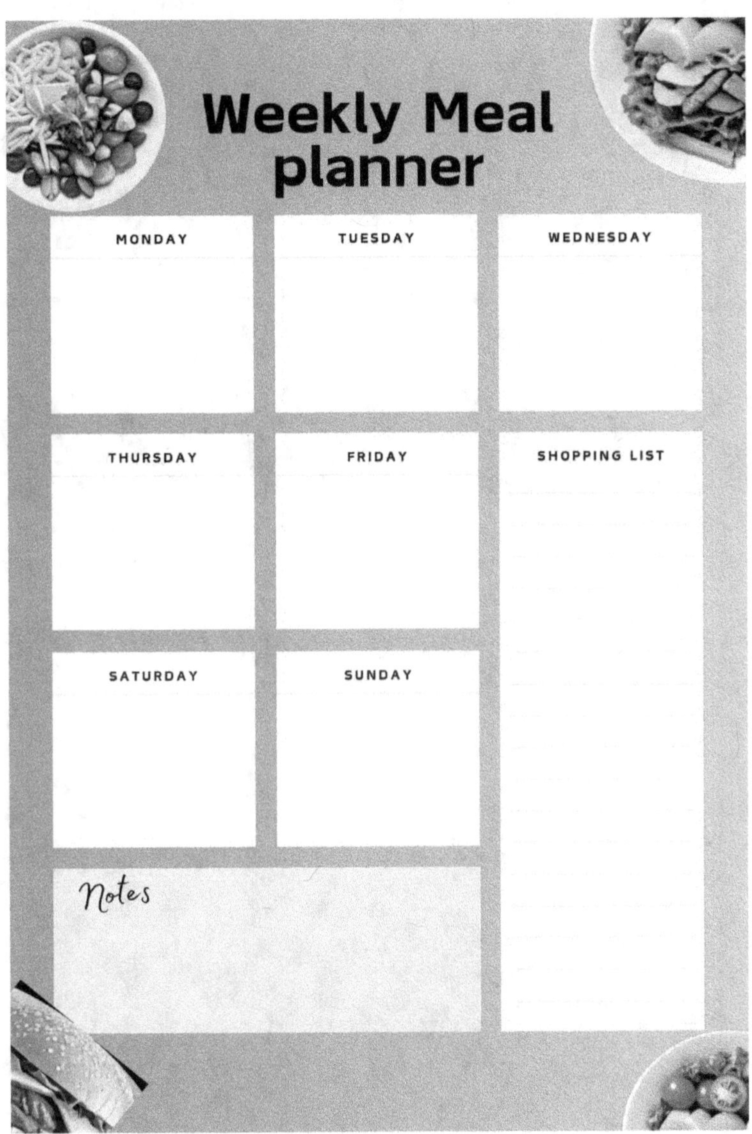

Weekly Meal
planner
MONDAY
TUESDAY
WEDNESDAY
THURSDAY
FRIDAY
SHOPPING LIST
SATURDAY
SUNDAY
Notes

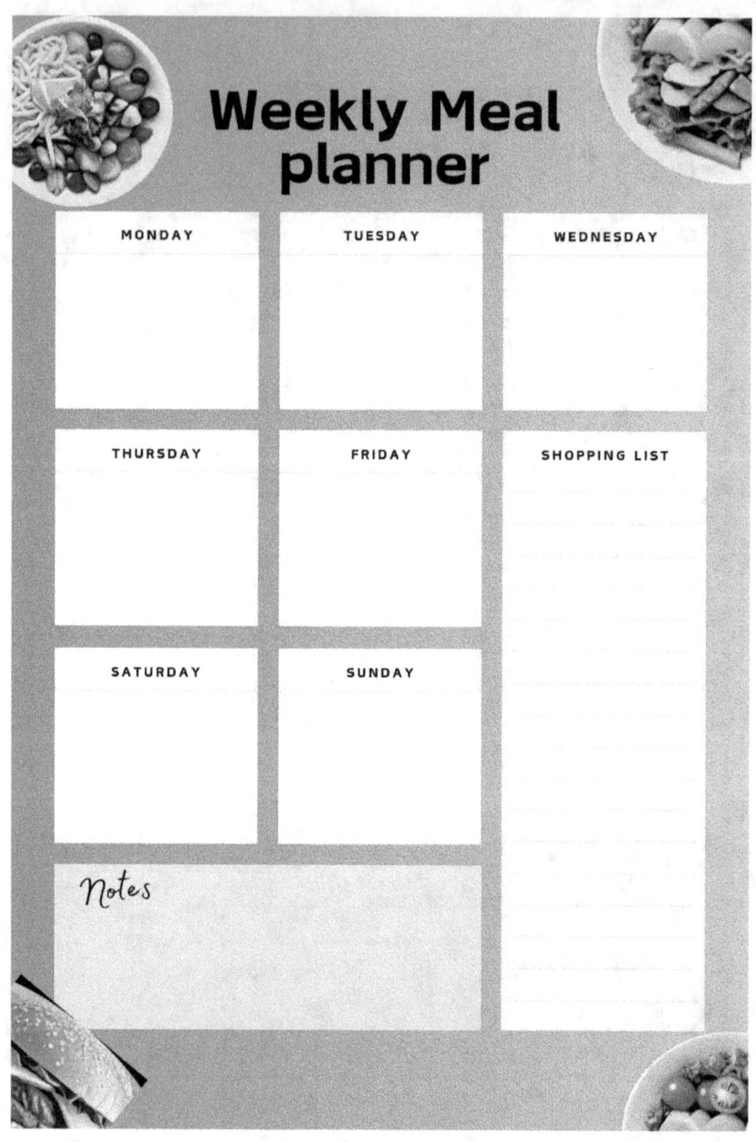

225

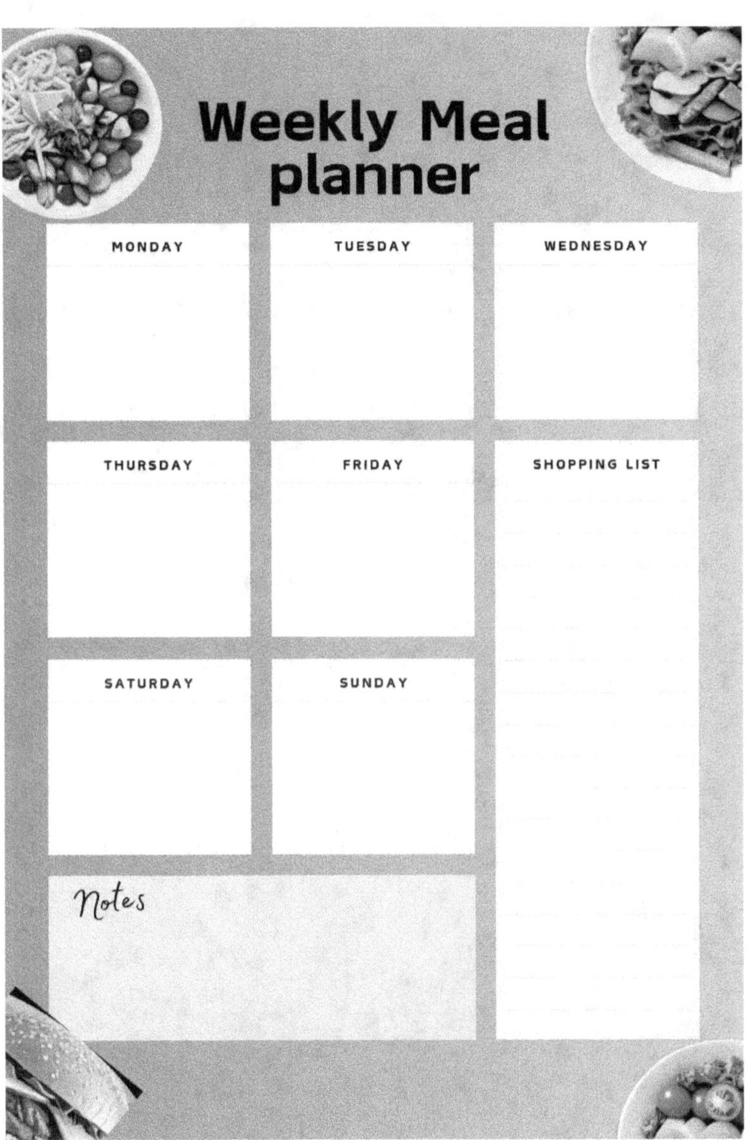

Weekly Meal planner
MONDAY
TUESDAY
WEDNESDAY
THURSDAY
FRIDAY
SHOPPING LIST
SATURDAY
SUNDAY
Notes

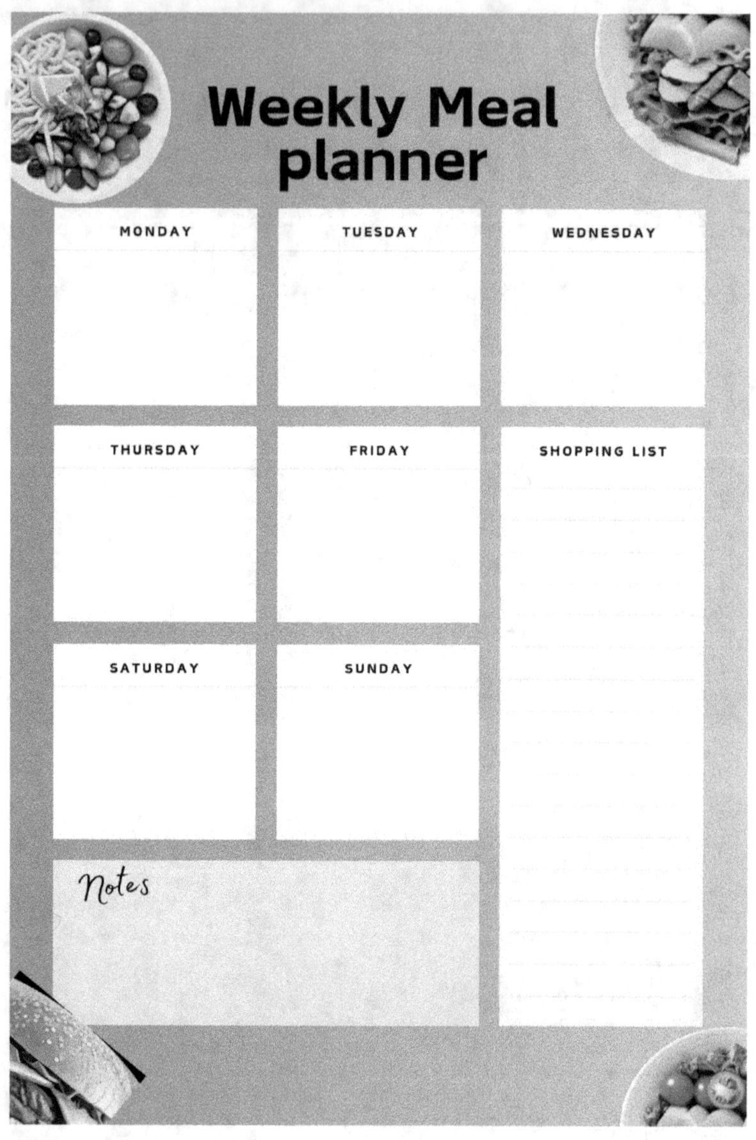

Weekly Meal planner
MONDAY
TUESDAY
WEDNESDAY
THURSDAY
FRIDAY
SHOPPING LIST
SATURDAY
SUNDAY
Notes

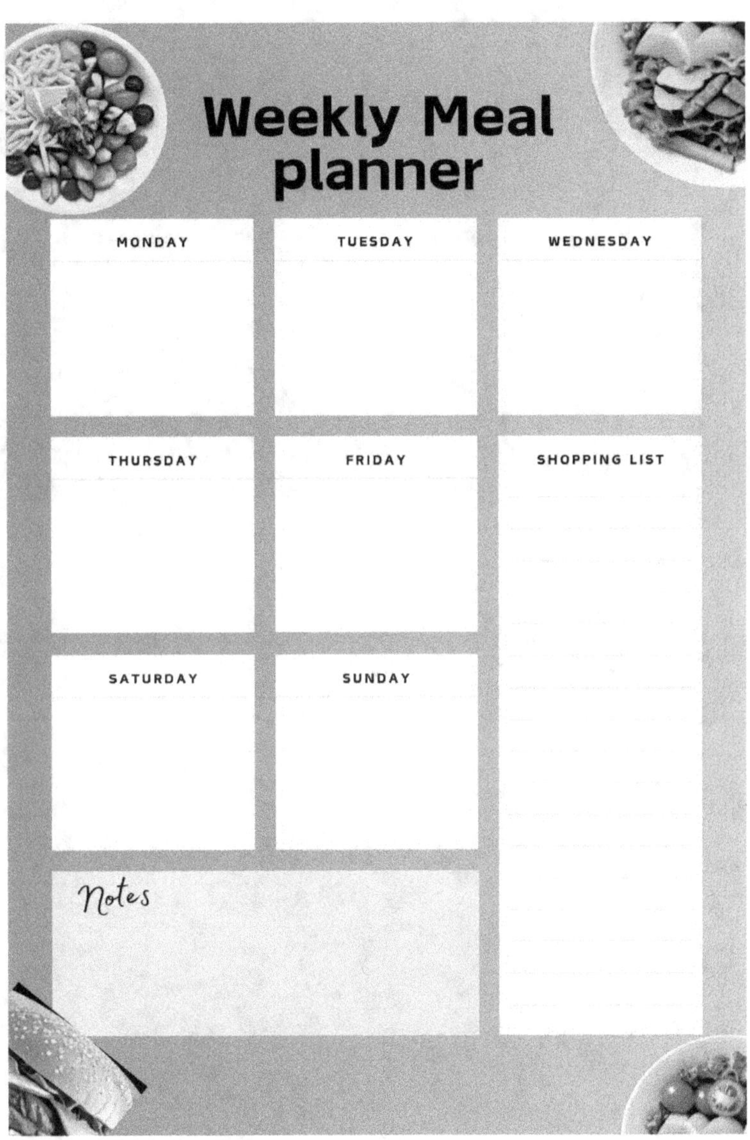

Weekly Meal planner
MONDAY
TUESDAY
WEDNESDAY
THURSDAY
FRIDAY
SHOPPING LIST
SATURDAY
SUNDAY
Notes

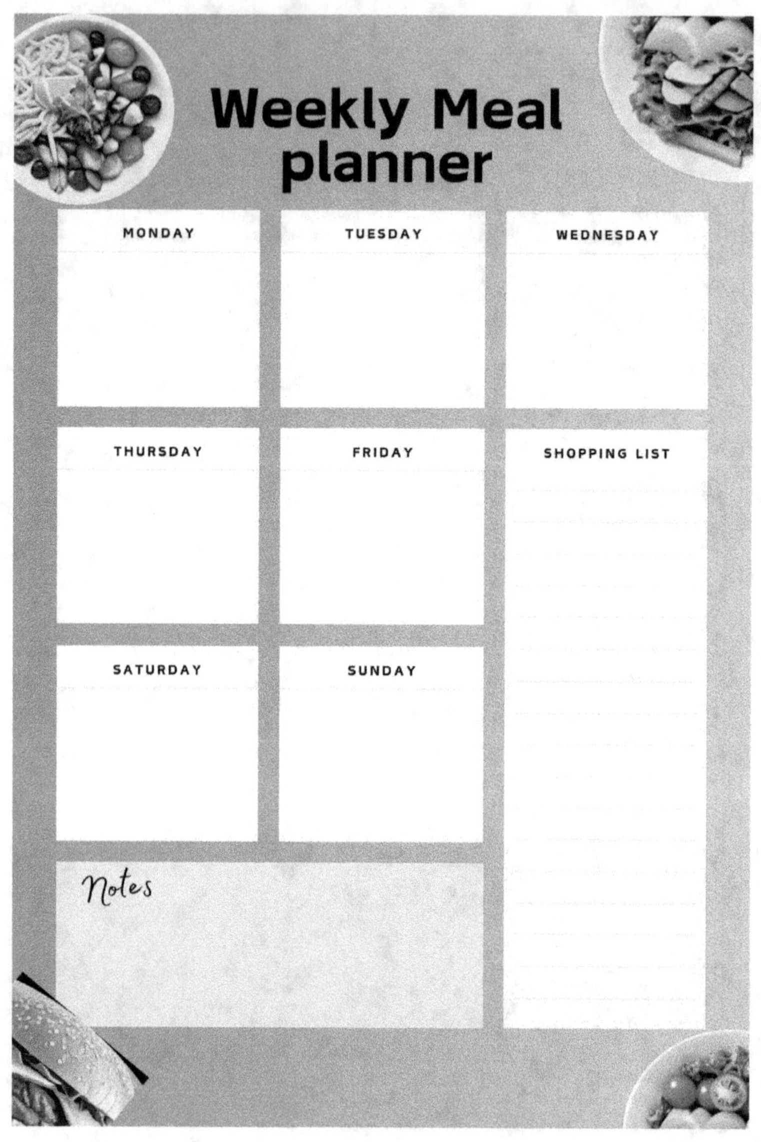

Weekly Meal
planner
MONDAY
TUESDAY
WEDNESDAY
THURSDAY
FRIDAY
SHOPPING LIST
SATURDAY
SUNDAY
Notes

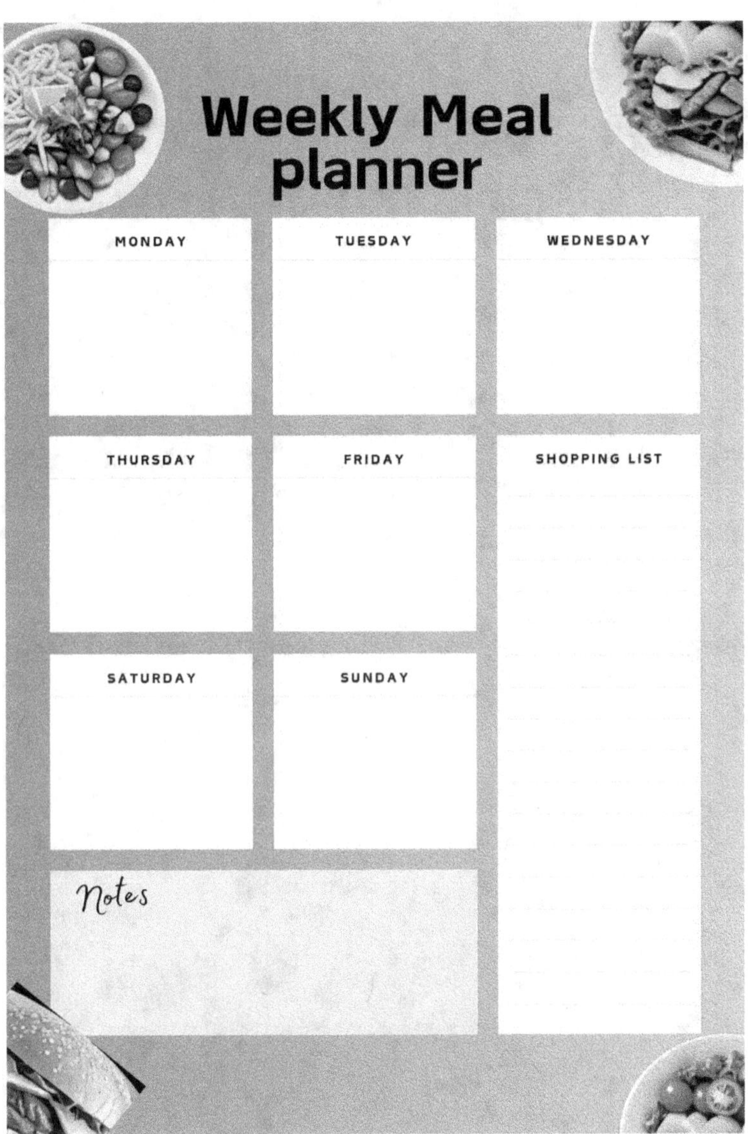

Weekly Meal
planner
MONDAY
TUESDAY
WEDNESDAY
THURSDAY
FRIDAY
SHOPPING LIST
SATURDAY
SUNDAY
Notes

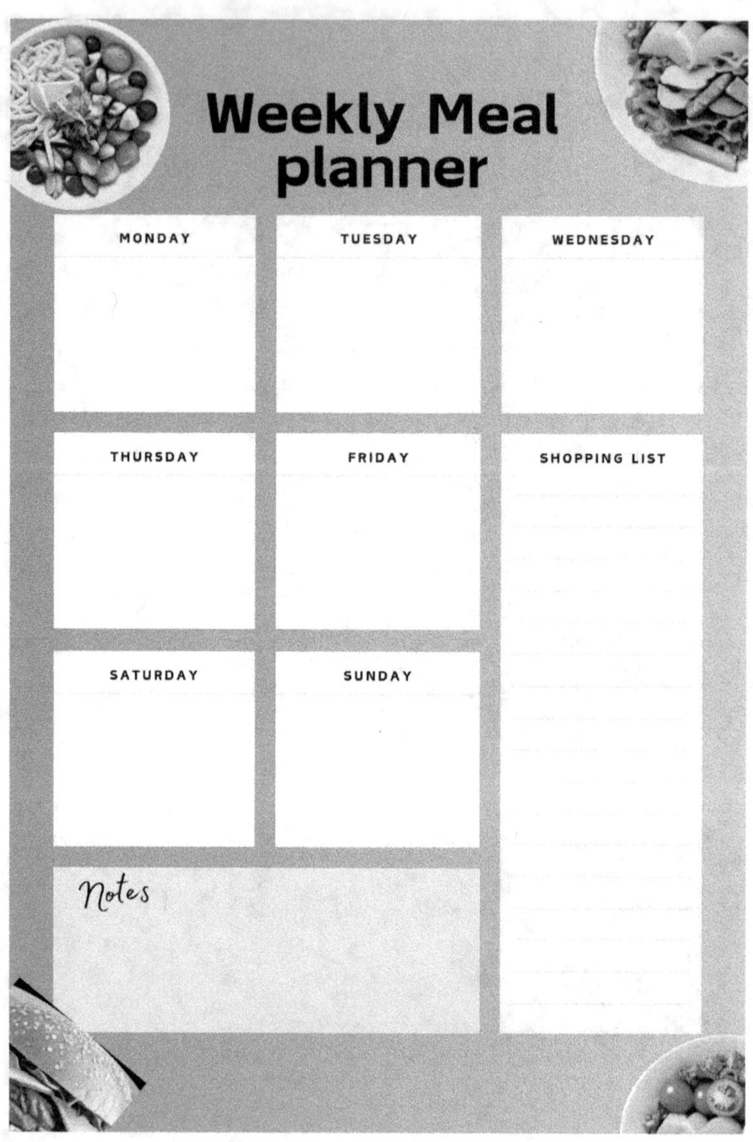

Weekly Meal planner
MONDAY
TUESDAY
WEDNESDAY
THURSDAY
FRIDAY
SHOPPING LIST
SATURDAY
SUNDAY
Notes

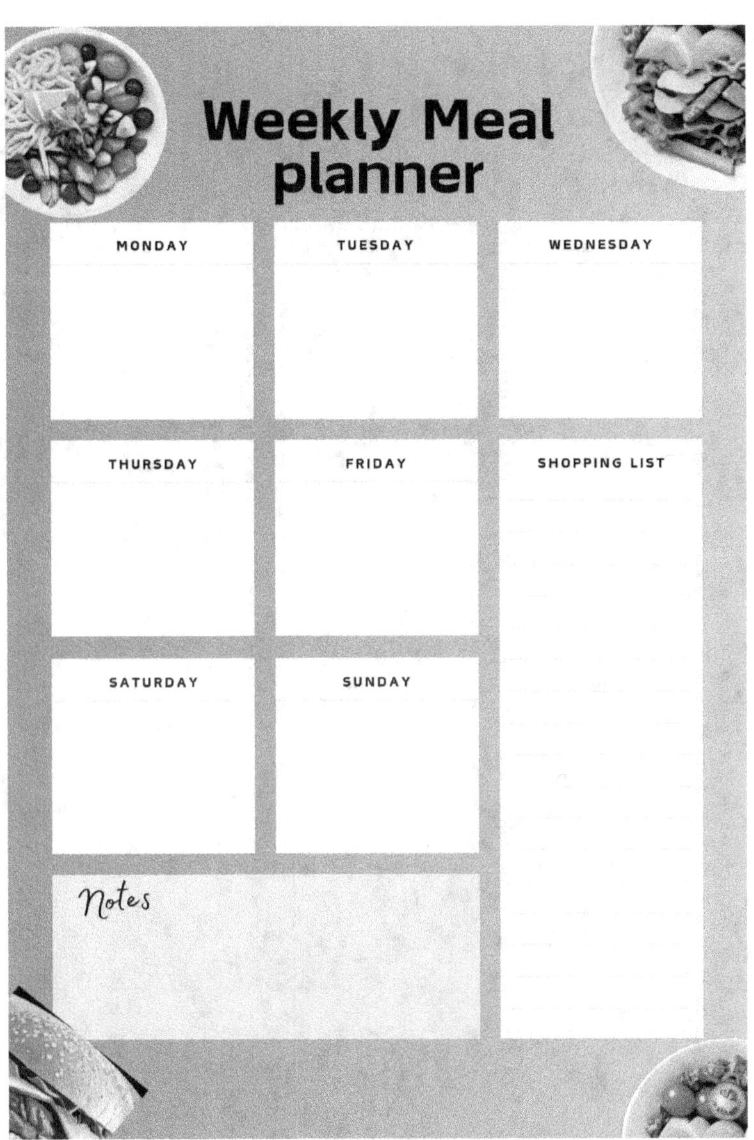

232

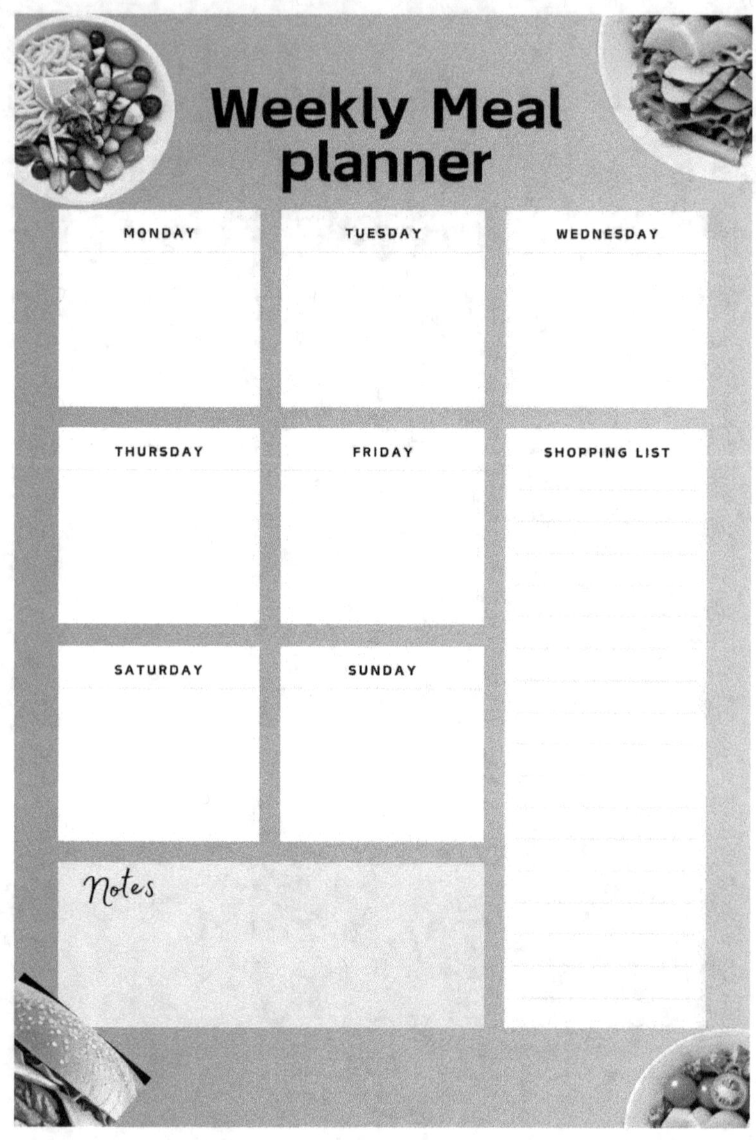

Weekly Meal planner
MONDAY
TUESDAY
WEDNESDAY
THURSDAY
FRIDAY
SHOPPING LIST
SATURDAY
SUNDAY
Notes

Example Weekly Meal Plan Template:

Monday:
- Breakfast: Greek Yogurt Parfait
- Lunch: Mediterranean Quinoa Salad
- Snack: Veggie Sticks with Hummus
- Dinner: Baked Salmon with Lemon and Herbs

Tuesday:
- Breakfast: Spinach and Feta Omelet
- Lunch: Grilled Chicken and Avocado Salad
- Snack: Almond Butter Energy Bites
- Dinner: Sweet Potato and Black Bean Tacos

Wednesday:
- Breakfast: Berry Antioxidant Smoothie
- Lunch: Tuna Salad Lettuce Wraps
- Snack: Apple Slices with Almond Butter
- Dinner: Chicken and Veggie Stir-Fry

Thursday:
- Breakfast: Chia Seed Pudding
- Lunch: Lentil and Spinach Salad
- Snack: Baked Kale Chips
- Dinner: Zucchini Noodles with Pesto

Friday:
- Breakfast: Avocado and Egg Toast
- Lunch: Roasted Beet and Goat Cheese Salad
- Snack: Greek Yogurt with Honey and Nuts
- Dinner: Beef and Broccoli Stir-Fry

Saturday:
- Breakfast: Almond Flour Pancakes
- Lunch: Quinoa and Black Bean Salad
- Snack: Dark Chocolate Almond Bark
- Dinner: Moroccan Chicken with Quinoa

Sunday:
- Breakfast: Sweet Potato Hash with Eggs
- Lunch: Vegan Buddha Bowl
- Snack: Cucumber and Smoked Salmon Bites
- Dinner: Garlic Herb Roasted Chicken

Tips for Using the Weekly Meal Plan Template:

1. Customize to Your Preferences: Adjust the meal plan based on your dietary preferences, allergies, and specific nutritional needs.

2. Plan for Leftovers: Cook larger portions for dinner and use the leftovers for lunch the next day.

3. Incorporate Variety: Rotate different recipes each week to keep your meals exciting and diverse.

4. Prep Ahead: Use the meal prep strategies in the next chapter to prepare ingredients in advance and make meal preparation easier.

Balanced Meal Ideas

A balanced meal contains a variety of nutrients that help sustain energy levels, promote hormone balance, and support overall health. Here are some balanced meal ideas that fit the Galveston Diet principles:

Breakfast:
- Protein-Packed Omelet: Eggs, spinach, mushrooms, and feta cheese.
- Flaxseed Banana Smoothie: Almond milk, banana, flaxseeds, and a handful of spinach.

Lunch:
- Grilled Chicken and Avocado Salad: Grilled chicken breast, mixed greens, avocado, cherry tomatoes, and a light vinaigrette.

- Quinoa and Black Bean Salad: Quinoa, black beans, corn, red bell pepper, and a lime-cilantro dressing.

Dinner:
- Salmon and Asparagus Salad: Grilled salmon, roasted asparagus, mixed greens, and a lemon-dill dressing.
- Turkey Meatballs in Tomato Sauce: Turkey meatballs simmered in homemade tomato sauce, served with zucchini noodles.

Snacks:
- Veggie Sticks with Hummus: Carrot sticks, celery sticks, and homemade hummus.
- Greek Yogurt with Honey and Nuts: Plain Greek yogurt topped with a drizzle of honey and a handful of nuts.

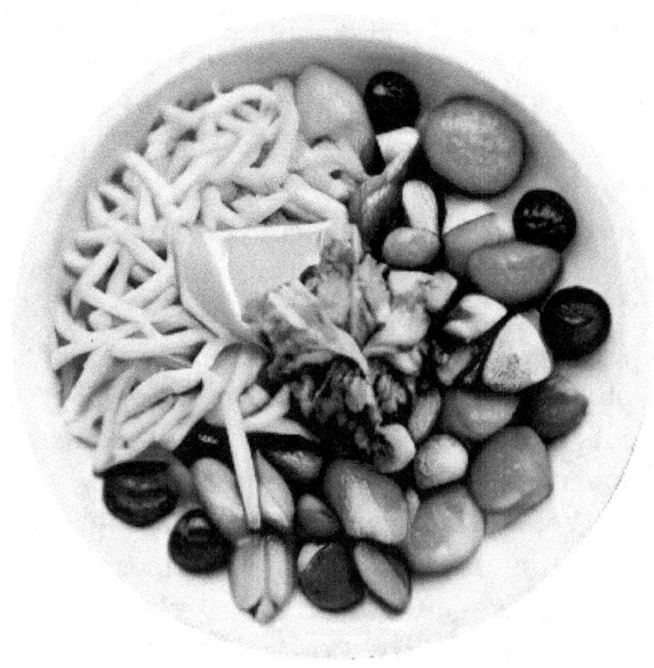

Chapter 11: Meal Prep Strategies for Success

Meal prep can be a game-changer in maintaining a healthy diet, especially when following the Galveston Diet. By dedicating a few hours each week to meal prep, you can ensure you have healthy meals and snacks ready to go, making it easier to stick to your nutrition goals.

Batch Cooking Tips

1. Cook in Bulk: Prepare large quantities of grains, proteins, and vegetables that can be used in multiple meals throughout the week.

2. Use Versatile Ingredients: Cook ingredients that can be used in various recipes, such as roasted chicken, quinoa, and roasted vegetables.

3. Invest in Quality Containers: Use airtight containers to store prepped food to maintain freshness and make reheating easier.

4. Label and Date: Label containers with the name of the dish and the date it was prepared to keep track of freshness.

Example Batch Cooking Plan:

- Proteins: Grill or bake a batch of chicken breasts, cook a pot of quinoa, and roast a tray of chickpeas.
- Vegetables: Roast a variety of vegetables such as sweet potatoes, carrots, and bell peppers.
- Grains: Cook a large pot of brown rice or quinoa.

Time-Saving Techniques

1. Plan Ahead: Create a meal plan and grocery list before heading to the store to ensure you have all necessary ingredients.
2. Prep Ingredients in Advance: Wash and chop vegetables, marinate proteins, and portion out snacks ahead of time.
3. Use a Slow Cooker or Instant Pot: These appliances can save time by cooking meals while you focus on other tasks.
4. Double Up Recipes: When cooking, make double the recipe and freeze half for future meals.

Storage and Reheating Tips

1. Proper Storage: Store prepped food in airtight containers in the refrigerator or freezer to maintain freshness.

2. Use Mason Jars: For salads and soups, use mason jars to keep ingredients fresh and make reheating easy.

3. Reheating Tips: Reheat meals on the stove or in the microwave, adding a splash of water or broth to prevent drying out.

4. Frozen Meals: Label frozen meals with the date and reheating instructions to make it easy to enjoy a home-cooked meal anytime.

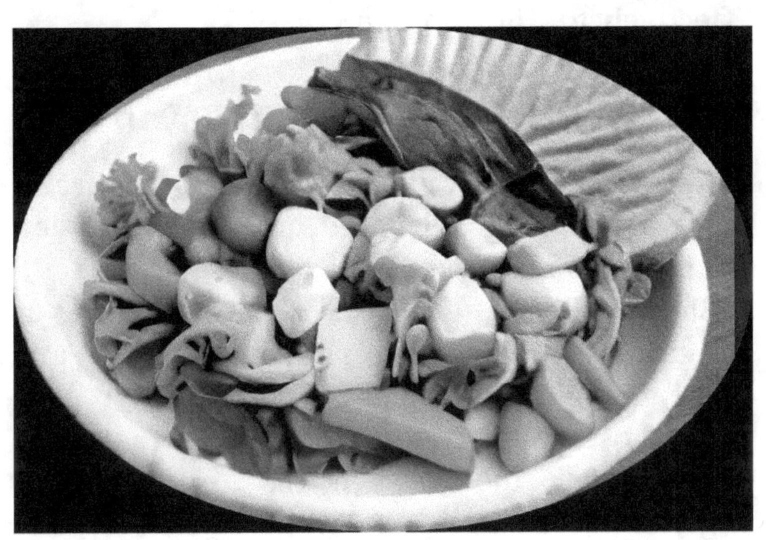

242

Chapter 12: Grocery Shopping Tips and Tricks

Grocery shopping can be overwhelming, but with the right strategies, it can be a straightforward and enjoyable process. Here's how to shop effectively for the Galveston Diet.

How to Shop for the Galveston Diet

1. Plan Your Meals: Create a weekly meal plan and make a shopping list based on the recipes you plan to prepare.

2. Shop the Perimeter: Focus on the outer aisles of the grocery store where fresh produce, meats, and dairy are typically located.

3. Choose Whole Foods: Opt for whole, unprocessed foods such as fresh fruits, vegetables, lean meats, and whole grains.

4. Buy in Bulk: Purchase bulk items like grains, nuts, and seeds to save money and ensure you always have essentials on hand.

Sample Grocery List for the Galveston Diet:

Produce:
- **Spinach**
- **Kale**
- **Avocados**
- **Berries**
- **Sweet potatoes**
- **Bell peppers**
- **Onions**
- **Garlic**
- **Zucchini**
- **Tomatoes**

Proteins:
- **Chicken breasts**
- **Salmon filets**
- **Ground turkey**
- **Eggs**
- **Greek yogurt**

Grains and Legumes:
- **Quinoa**
- **Brown rice**
- **Lentils**

- Black beans
- Chickpeas

Healthy Fats:
- Olive oil
- Almond butter
- Nuts and seeds

Other Essentials:
- Spices (turmeric, cumin, oregano)
- Herbs (cilantro, parsley)
- Low-sodium vegetable broth
- Canned diced tomatoes

Reading Nutrition Labels

Understanding nutrition labels is crucial for making informed food choices. Here are some key points to consider:

1. Serving Size: Check the serving size to understand the nutritional information relative to how much you actually consume.
2. Calories: Consider the calorie content in relation to your daily needs.
3. Macronutrients: Look at the amounts of fat, carbohydrates, and protein. Aim for a balance that fits your dietary goals.

4. Ingredients List: Choose products with a short, recognizable ingredients list. Avoid items with added sugars, artificial ingredients, and preservatives.

5. Fiber and Sugar: Opt for foods high in fiber and low in added sugars.

Example Nutrition Label Breakdown:

Product: Greek Yogurt
- Serving Size: 1 cup (8 oz)
- Calories: 150
- Total Fat: 3g
- Saturated Fat: 1g
- Cholesterol: 10mg
- Sodium: 60mg
- Total Carbohydrates: 9g
- Dietary Fiber: 0g
- Sugars: 6g
- Protein: 20g
- Ingredients: Pasteurized milk, live active cultures.

By incorporating these meal planning, prep, and grocery shopping strategies, you can streamline your approach to healthy eating and make the Galveston Diet a sustainable and enjoyable part of your lifestyle. Remember, consistency is key, and planning ahead will help you stay on track and achieve your health goals.

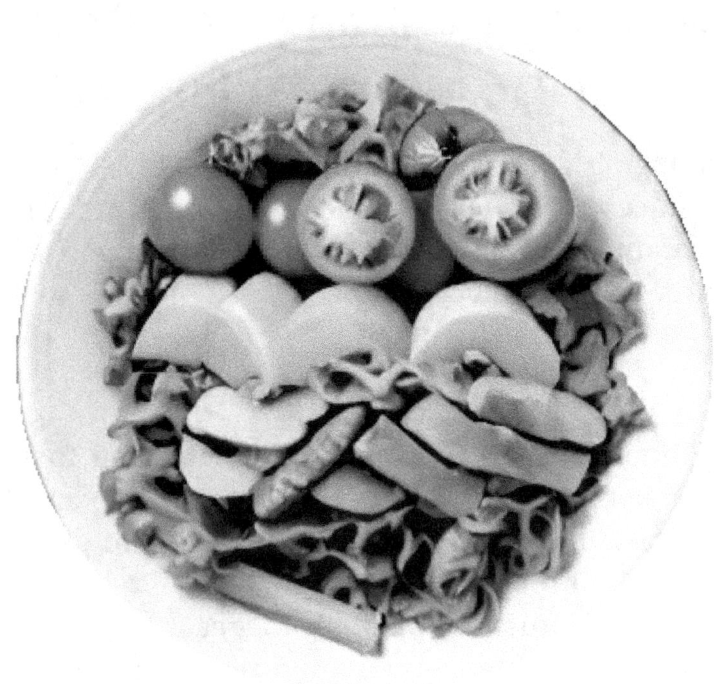

Chapter 13: Stress Management and Self-Care for Hormone Balance

Managing stress and incorporating self-care practices are crucial components of maintaining hormone balance and overall well-being while following the Galveston Diet.

Meditation Techniques

1. Mindfulness Meditation: Sit quietly and focus on your breath. When thoughts arise, acknowledge them without judgment and gently return your focus to your breath.

2. Guided Imagery: Listen to recordings that guide you through visualizing calming scenes or positive outcomes.

3. Body Scan Meditation: Focus on each part of your body, starting from your toes to your head, noticing any sensations without trying to change them.

4. Mantra Meditation: Repeat a calming word or phrase silently or aloud to anchor your mind and reduce stress.

Stress-Reducing Activities

1. Deep Breathing: Practice deep breathing exercises to calm your nervous system.
2. Nature Walks: Spend time outdoors in nature, which can reduce cortisol levels and improve mood.
3. Art or Creative Expression: Engage in activities like painting, drawing, or playing music to relax and unwind.
4. Journaling: Write about your thoughts and feelings to gain clarity and reduce stress.

Self-Care Routines

1. Daily Routine: Establish a consistent daily routine that includes regular meals, exercise, and relaxation.
2. Quality Sleep: Prioritize getting enough restful sleep each night to support hormone balance and overall health.
3. Healthy Boundaries: Set boundaries to protect your time and energy, and learn to say no when necessary.

4. **Social Connection:** Nurture relationships with friends and loved ones for emotional support and connection.

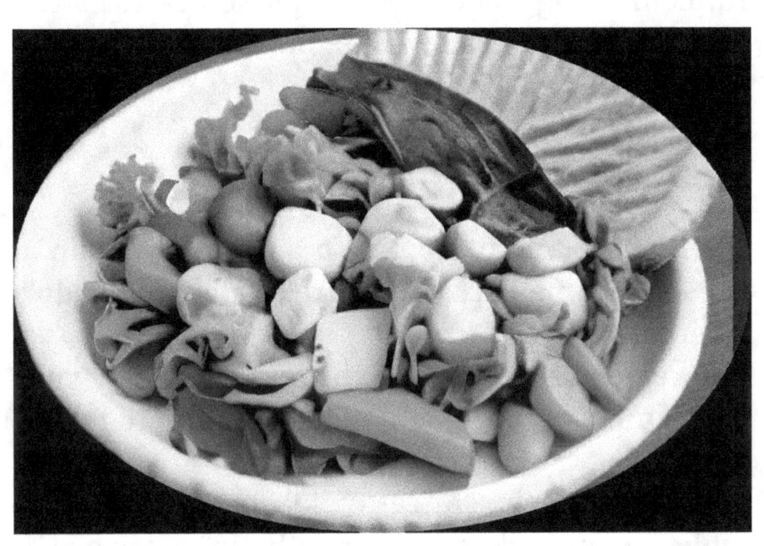

Chapter 14: Getting Enough Sleep for Weight Loss and Vitality

Adequate sleep is essential for hormone regulation, metabolism, and overall vitality. Implementing good sleep hygiene practices can enhance your overall well-being and support your weight loss goals.

Sleep Hygiene Tips

1. Establish a Routine: Go to bed and wake up at the same time each day to regulate your body's internal clock.

2. Create a Relaxing Environment: Keep your bedroom cool, dark, and quiet to promote restful sleep.

3. Limit Screen Time: Avoid screens (phones, tablets, computers) at least an hour before bed as the blue light can interfere with melatonin production.

4. Avoid Stimulants: Limit caffeine and nicotine intake, especially in the afternoon and evening.

5. Wind Down: Develop a relaxing bedtime routine such as reading a book, taking a warm bath, or practicing gentle yoga.

Evening Routine Ideas

1. Herbal Tea: Enjoy a cup of chamomile or lavender tea, known for their calming properties.
2. Light Stretching: Perform gentle stretching exercises to release tension and prepare your body for sleep.
3. Mindfulness Practice: Practice meditation or deep breathing to quiet the mind before bedtime.
4. Journaling: Write down any worries or thoughts to clear your mind before sleep.

Importance of Rest and Recovery

1. Muscle Repair: Sleep allows your muscles to recover and repair from daily activities and workouts.
2. Cognitive Function: Adequate sleep supports memory, concentration, and overall cognitive function.
3. Hormone Regulation: Sleep plays a crucial role in regulating hormones that control appetite, metabolism, and stress response.

Chapter 15: Exercise and Movement for Sustainable Weight Loss

Regular exercise and movement are essential for maintaining a healthy weight, improving mood, and supporting overall well-being.

Integrating Workouts

1. Cardiovascular Exercise: Engage in activities such as brisk walking, jogging, cycling, or swimming to improve heart health and burn calories.
2. Strength Training: Incorporate resistance exercises using weights, resistance bands, or bodyweight exercises to build muscle and boost metabolism.
3. Flexibility Training: Practice stretching or yoga to improve flexibility, reduce stiffness, and enhance relaxation.

Yoga and Mindfulness Practices

1. Yoga: Attend yoga classes or follow online videos to improve flexibility, strength, and mindfulness.

2. Mindful Movement: Practice tai chi or qigong, which combines slow, deliberate movements with deep breathing for relaxation and stress reduction.

Strength Training Tips

1. Progressive Overload: Gradually increase the weight or resistance to continue challenging your muscles and promote growth.
2. Compound Exercises: Incorporate compound movements like squats, deadlifts, and push-ups that engage multiple muscle groups simultaneously.
3. Rest Days: Allow time for muscle recovery by alternating between different muscle groups and incorporating rest days into your routine.

By incorporating these lifestyle and self-care practices, including stress management techniques, prioritizing sleep, and engaging in regular exercise, you can enhance the benefits of the Galveston Diet and support your journey towards sustainable weight loss and improved vitality. Remember to listen to your body, make adjustments as needed, and enjoy the process of nurturing your overall health and well-being.

Chapter 16: Customizing the Galveston Diet for Your Needs

Tailoring the Galveston Diet to suit individual preferences and health goals is essential for long-term success. This chapter explores how you can personalize your meal plan and adjust various aspects of the diet to meet your specific needs.

Personalizing Your Meal Plan

1. Assessing Dietary Preferences: Identify foods you enjoy and incorporate them into your meal plan while adhering to the principles of the Galveston Diet.

2. Allergies and Intolerances: Modify recipes to accommodate allergies or intolerances without compromising nutritional balance.

3. Cultural Considerations: Adapt recipes to align with cultural dietary practices and preferences.

Adjusting Potions and Ingredients

1. Portion Control Strategies: Learn portion sizes appropriate for your individual calorie needs and weight loss goals.

2. Ingredient Substitutions: Substitute ingredients to accommodate dietary restrictions or preferences while maintaining nutrient density.

Chapter 17: Troubleshooting Common Challenges

Navigating obstacles is an inevitable part of any health journey. This chapter addresses common challenges that individuals may encounter while following the Galveston Diet and provides practical solutions to overcome them.

Overcoming Plateaus

1. Reassessing Caloric Intake: Adjust your calorie intake based on changes in weight and activity level to break through weight loss plateaus.

2. Increasing Physical Activity: Incorporate additional physical activity or modify exercise routines to boost metabolism and promote fat loss.

3. Varying Meal Options: Introduce variety into your meal plan to prevent metabolic adaptation and encourage continued weight loss.

Managing Cravings

1. Identifying Triggers: Recognize triggers that lead to cravings and develop strategies to manage them effectively.

2. Healthy Alternatives: Substitute unhealthy cravings with nutritious alternatives that satisfy cravings without derailing your diet.

3. Mindful Eating: Practice mindful eating techniques to become more aware of hunger and satiety cues, reducing the likelihood of succumbing to cravings.

Staying Motivated

1. Setting Realistic Goals: Establish achievable short-term and long-term goals to maintain motivation throughout your health journey.

2. Tracking Progress: Monitor your progress by tracking measurements, weight, and other relevant metrics to celebrate achievements and stay motivated.

3. Seeking Support: Engage with a supportive community, friends, or family members who can encourage and motivate you during challenging times.

Chapter 18: Maintaining Weight Loss and Hormone Balance Long-Term

Sustainable health and well-being require long-term commitment and lifestyle adjustments. This chapter provides strategies to sustain weight loss, support hormone balance, and foster overall health in the long term.

Long-term Meal Planning

1. Weekly Meal Planning: Continue planning and preparing meals in advance to maintain healthy eating habits and avoid impulsive food choices.
2. Batch Cooking: Incorporate batch cooking techniques to save time and ensure nutritious meals are readily available throughout the week.

Tips for Dining Out

1. Menu Selection: Choose restaurants with healthier menu options that align with the principles of the Galveston Diet.
2. Meal Preparation: Plan ahead by reviewing restaurant menus online and making informed choices before arriving.

3. Portion Control: Practice portion control by sharing meals or requesting smaller portions when dining out.

Handling Social Situations

1. Communicating Dietary Needs: Clearly communicate your dietary preferences and restrictions to friends, family, and hosts when attending social gatherings.

2. Bringing Your Own Dish: Offer to bring a nutritious dish to social events to ensure there are healthy options available.

3. Balancing Indulgences: Enjoy occasional indulgences while maintaining overall balance and moderation in your diet.

Conclusion

Congratulations on Taking the First Step Towards Transforming Your Health!

Embarking on the Galveston Diet is a significant step towards achieving sustainable weight loss, hormone balance, and vitality. Reflect on your journey and celebrate your accomplishments.

Reflecting on Your Journey

1. Achievements: Acknowledge the progress you've made towards improving your health and well-being.
2. Challenges: Reflect on challenges you've overcome and the lessons learned along the way.
3. Personal Growth: Consider how adopting healthier habits has positively impacted your life and outlook on health.

Staying Motivated and Inspired

1. Setting New Goals: Continue setting new health goals to maintain momentum and continue your journey towards lifelong health.

2. Inspiration: Draw inspiration from success stories, motivational resources, and supportive communities to stay motivated.

3. Self-Care: Prioritize self-care practices that nourish your mind, body, and spirit throughout your health journey.

The Next Steps to Lifelong Health

1. Continued Learning: Stay informed about nutrition, health trends, and scientific research to continue making informed choices.

2. Adaptation: Be open to adapting your diet and lifestyle as needed to support changing health needs and goals.

3. Consistency: Maintain consistency in healthy habits while allowing flexibility to enjoy life's moments.

Thoughts and Encouragement

Embrace the journey of transforming your health with the Galveston Diet as a foundation for lifelong well-being. Remember, every positive choice you make contributes to your overall health and vitality.

This comprehensive conclusion and advanced topics section provide practical advice and encouragement to help readers customize their approach to the Galveston Diet, troubleshoot challenges, and maintain long-term success in achieving health and wellness goals.

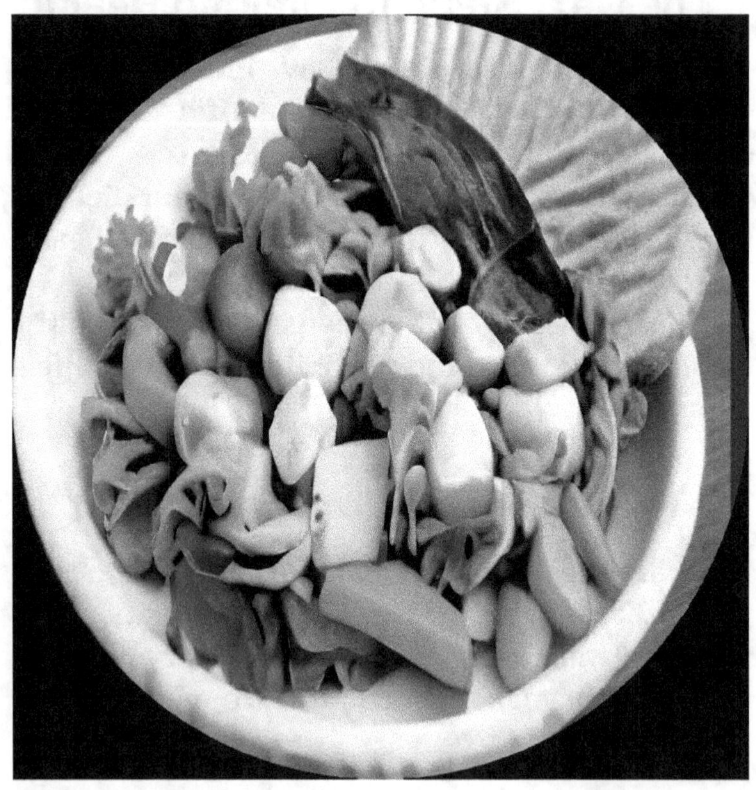

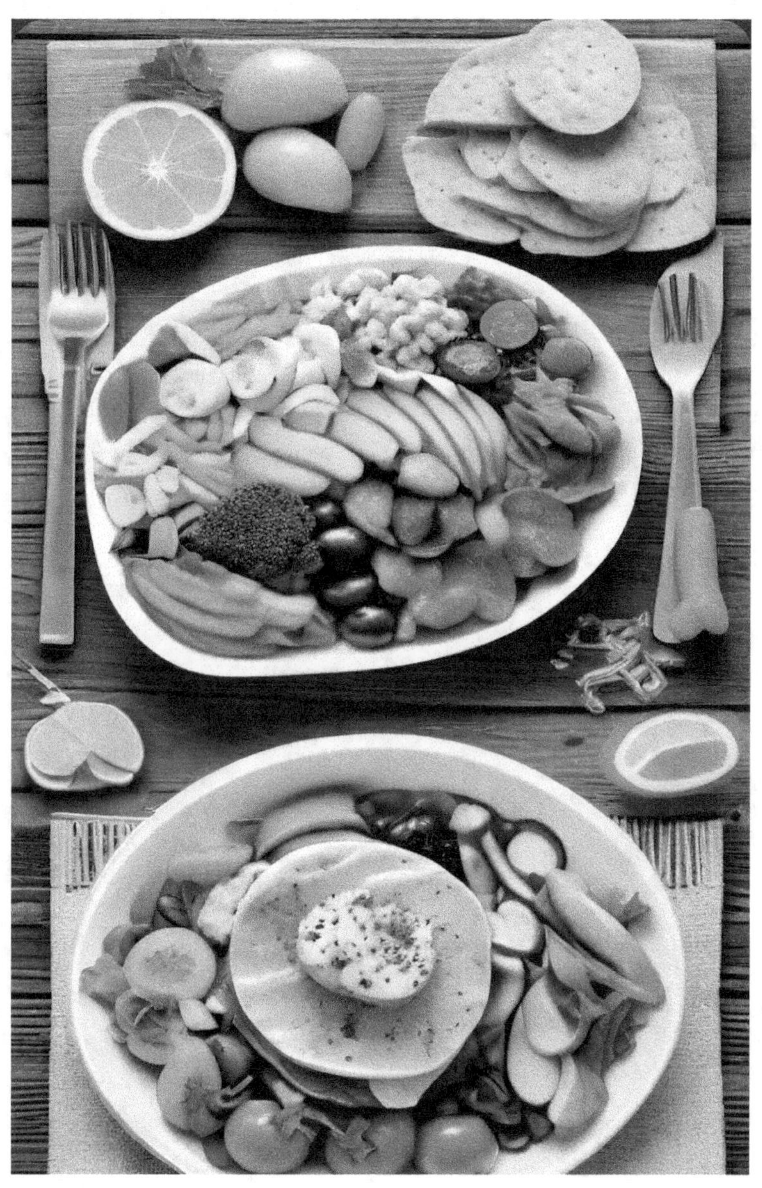

www.ingramcontent.com/pod-product-compliance
Lightning Source LLC
Chambersburg PA
CBHW051551250726

48653CB00004BA/1101